THE TRUTH ABOUT
AIR ELECTRICITY
& HEALTH

A guide on the use of air ionization and other natural
approaches for 21st century health issues.

Rosalind Tan

Rosalind Tan shows an authority over her subject that only comes with much research, work and passion. Once I started reading this work I couldn't stop, as I understood the importance of this subject. She presents it in a very engaging and readable manner.

She shows us very clearly why we should, with all doubt removed, pay much closer attention to the quality of the air we breathe. In a world of failing health and this becomes required reading for any parent wanting to create a safe, nurturing environment for their family.

I intend to make this work available to all my clients seeking a healthier life."

Dr Tim Errington BSC DC

Total Health Chiropractic, Singapore

For book orders, email orders@traffordpublishing.com.sg

Most Trafford Singapore titles are also available at major online book retailers.

Printed in Singapore.

ISBN: 978-1-4907-0059-5 (sc)
ISBN: 978-1-4907-0060-1 (hc)
ISBN: 978-1-4907-0061-8 (e)

Trafford rev. 12/20/2013

Trafford www.traffordpublishing.com.sg
Singapore
toll-free: 800 101 2656 (Singapore)
Fax: 800 101 2656 (Singapore)

CONTENTS

INTRODUCTION

"Negative ions are the vitamins of the air."
—Dr. E. R. Holiday

There are endless case histories of people who have reversed their poor health condition by simply moving to the mountains or to the sea. Sanitariums were traditionally built for the treatment of tuberculosis in the European Alps and doctors worldwide have advocated a 'change of air' for their patients.

Pale, frail and only twenty-five, Martha Rebentisch, against all medical advice, moved into the woods to start her new life. Martha had tuberculosis which, before the days of antibiotics, was the number one killer in America. In three and a half years in several healing centers, Martha had undergone three painful operations which failed to cure her of her disease. Now, instead of going through yet more surgery, she responded to an ad:

> WANTED: To get in touch with some invalid who is not improving, and who wants to go into the woods for the summer.

Martha Rebentisch's book *Healing Woods* chronicles her miraculous recovery from TB in the Adirondack Mountains where she spent many happy years enjoying the wildlife and the curative powers of the Adirondack woods' air.

Some years earlier, Dr Hermann Brehmer, a German physician, had advocated an abundance of mountain fresh air and good nutrition for the treatment of tuberculosis. While still a botany student, he was diagnosed with tuberculosis, but he found himself cured of the ravaging disease after his retreat to the Himalayas in search of a healthier climate. Dr Brehmer subsequently wrote a thesis entitled *Tuberculosis is a Curable Disease* and founded the first German sanatorium for the systematic open-air treatment of tuberculosis.

Weak and without any hope of recovery, New York City doctor Edward Livingston Trudeau came to the Adirondack Mountains in 1873 to die quietly in a more pleasant environment. Amazingly, the doctor recovered from his supposedly incurable disease, living on fresh mountain air.

What is it about air? Why should the air in the hills or by the sea be better for us than the air inside the cities?

The answer lies in a tiny electrically charged air molecule known as a **negative ion.**

Certain environments are invigorating due to the abundance of negative ions in the air. Such environments include waterfall areas, pine forests, or the seashore where the surf crashes on the rocks.

Alpine and mountain areas more than 5,000 feet above sea level also have an enriched negative ion atmosphere, which explains the feeling of well-being. In these environments you will experience a level of energy that is vastly different from your energy when sitting at a desk in the office in front of a display screen.

Thousands of published reports have demonstrated the clear link between air ions and the health of living organisms. University and medical research throughout the world verifies that an abundance of negative ions in the air has a positive effect on our health and wellbeing.

However, when nature or man meddles with air electricity and causes an overdose of positive ions in the ambient air, discomfort, misery and illness prevail.

In general, exposure to an abundance of negative ions can:

- Improve respiratory conditions such as asthma and allergies,
- Enable us to live longer,
- Cure depression and general lethargy,
- Prevent migraine headaches,
- Improve our sleep,
- Enable faster recovery from surgery,
- Enable faster healing from burns,
- Give us that feeling of "wellbeing" that is enjoyed by being in nature,
- Decrease the effects of ADHD and autism in our children,
- Improve our ability to focus and learn.

A lack of negative ions and too many positive ions can:

- Undermine the body's immune system
- Cause our bodies and minds to feel stressed and agitated,
- Exacerbate allergies, asthma and respiratory ills,
- Cause irritation and bad temperedness,
- Cause migraine headaches,
- Cause mental illness such as depression, anxiety and hyperactivity,
- Make our minds fuzzy and unable to gain clarity,
- Leave us feeling exhausted and tired.

Of course, we cannot all live in the mountains or by the sea! But we can artificially create more negative ions in the air we breathe.

This book

This book tells you of the harmful effects of modern day living in polluted cities on your health and the health of your children. The chapters explain how a combination of bad air quality and other factors such as chemicals in modern foodstuffs has led to serious physical and mental health problems.

The chapters describe how you can work to overcome these problems, by a healthier diet and lifestyle and by purifying the air that you breathe. The chapters provide a series of steps to follow towards a better future.

As you read this book, you will learn about negative ions, how they are produced in nature, and what an increase in negative ions can do for your health. You will also learn how we can increase the number of negative ions artificially in our immediate environment, even in offices and homes in polluted cities.

Although scientists have known of the benefits of negative ions for decades, there has been little education or publicity on the power that ionization has, on how negative ions support and improve mammalian life and on how they can cure many of our physical and mental ills.

Once you have read this book, you will understand that you can significantly make a difference to the health and wellbeing of your family by simply restoring the air electricity of your home and workplace.

CHAPTER 1

Why Air Electricity is Essential to our Life and Well-Being

"Nerve Force contains much of its power in the breath."
—Yoga Sutras

From Benjamin Franklin's theories of electrical energy of the air, which led to the invention of the lightning conductor, to the cumulative work of research scientists all over the world, it has been shown that air electricity comes from electrically charged molecules of gas called **ions**.

We live in an ocean of air and each of us is required to breathe in at least ten thousand liters of air every twenty-four hours just to maintain life in our bodies. Unbeknown to us all, we are breathing in minute charges of electricity all the time. Ions form only a small part of the air we breathe but it is the most important part.

What is an ion?

All matter, whether solid, liquid or gaseous, is made up of molecules. Each molecule consists of a dense core comprised of sub-atomic particles including positively charged protons. The core is surrounded by rapidly orbiting negatively-charged electrons. A normal passive molecule of air has the same number of protons and electrons, making it electrically neutral. This normal, electrically neutral molecule is said to be "stable" or "in equilibrium".

However, because an electron is 1800 times lighter than a proton, the electron is easily displaced by external forces. When an electron is detached from its orbiting path around an air molecule, the molecule has an imbalanced ratio of charges with a net positive charge. It is now a positive ion. The detached electron can enter into orbit in another molecule resulting in the molecule having more negative than positive charges. This becomes a negative ion.

In short, an **ion** is a molecule that has gained or lost an electron. A **negative ion** is an air molecule that has gained an electron. A positive ion is one that has lost an electron.

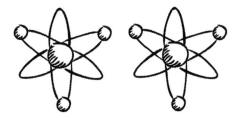

NEUTRAL ATOMS

Ions are formed when an electron is

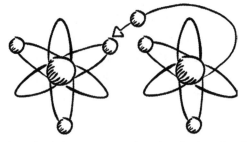

detached from a neutral molecule (or atom)

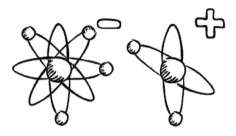

NEGATIVE IONS   POSITIVE IONS

The molecule losing an electron becomes a positive ion and the molecule gaining an electron becomes a negative ion

There are 27 thousand trillion stable molecules in every cubic centimeter of air but the number of ions varies, depending on the condition of the environment. In clean, open, country air we can expect about 1000 to 2000 ions per *cubic* centimeter. This is reduced to only a few hundred in a polluted environment or an enclosed, ill-ventilated, air-conditioned room.

There are both positive and negative ions in the air, but the negative ions are what give us the "feel-good" factor. More than just a feeling, negative ions stimulate and energize, and also destroy airborne bacteria and mold spores. This provides a possible explanation for the lack of fungus and mosses in pine forests—air-borne spores are destroyed by the high concentration of negative ions in the air of the pine forests.

Ions in nature

Our sun is made up mostly of hydrogen atoms. Helium is the second most plentiful element in the sun. The sun's energy is generated by what is known as the proton-proton nuclear chain reaction in which hydrogen is converted into helium and then back again.

This process produces the heat that sustains life on Earth, but also showers our planet with positive ions of hydrogen as a by-product.

In nature, everything is balanced. The earth, in its wisdom, responds to the bombardment of positive ions from the sun by producing negative ions through the breaking down of naturally occurring radium in the earth's crust to radon gas. This natural radiation causes oxygen ions to be formed.

The single charged molecule, called the primary ion, has the tendency to aggregate around airborne water droplets forming clusters of about six to eight molecules. These are regarded as small ions which are biologically effective. Small ions, when ingested, enhance the functionality of living systems, providing a sense of wellbeing.

The clustering behavior of air ions continues and small ions quickly grow to become intermediate and large ions, which are clusters of between fifty to several hundred molecules.

The decay of small ions into large ions is particularly rampant where there are vast amounts of airborne particulate matter, both man-made pollutants and natural dust and pollens. It is known that large clusters are of no biological significance to living organisms. In other words, they are not 'ingestible'.

The size of ions is measured by their mobility in an electrical field using an atmospheric ion analyzer. Small air ions are very active and they move around at great speed. Small air ions have a mobility range of $1\text{-}2\text{cm}^2/\text{Vs}$. Medium to large negative ions are sluggish and slow-moving.

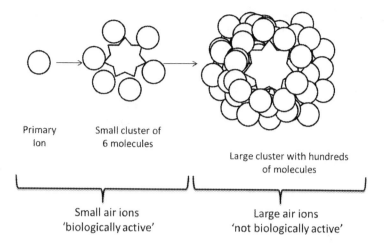

| Primary Ion | Small cluster of 6 molecules | Large cluster with hundreds of molecules |

Small air ions 'biologically active' | Large air ions 'not biologically active'

Primary ions usually form small clusters of 6-8 which is biologically active. Ions will cluster in much greater numbers around airborne particulate matter and these 'large ions' are biologically inactive.

Because the Earth is negatively charged, negative ions are propelled into the atmosphere and positive ions are drawn like a magnet to the surface area.

Normal air electricity has an ion balance of five small positive ions to four small negative ions and it is in this natural ion ratio that life exists and thrives. Studies and experience have shown that a change in this ratio in favor of positive ions is harmful, while an overdose of negative ions has curative properties.

The forces of nature also produce both negative and positive ions in abundance. High levels of negative air ions are created by lightning, cosmic rays, UV light and the natural process of photosynthesis carried out by green plants.

The shearing forces of water droplets, known as the Lenard effect, also create massive amounts of negative ions. This accounts for the euphoric feeling we experience after a heavy downpour, in waterfall areas or by the seaside. Friction between water and air causes electrons to be displaced and these fly free, forming negative ions while the heavier positive charges fall with the water droplets. Negative ions are dispersed into the air and we breathe them in.

Niagara Falls is lauded as the most impressive natural negative ion generator in the world, where there are more than 100 000 negative ions per cubic centimeter of air. That is why it has become a popular wellness destination attracting visitors from all parts of the world. To a lesser extent, man-made fountains and even the bathroom shower also have beneficial effects.

How it all started

Born in 1898 in the USA, Dr Clarence Hansell was a research engineer who investigated the properties of air. The biological effects of ionized air came to his attention in 1932, when he noticed that the moods of one of his colleagues changed drastically depending on whether negative or positive ions were being produced by the electrostatic generator next to where he was seated. When the ions were negative, his colleague was happy and upbeat, but when the ions were positive, he appeared to be ill-tempered, depressed and down in the mouth.

Dr Hansell researched negative ions throughout his life and his work on negative ion therapy for relieving depression is supported by current scientific studies.

Dr Hansell was not the only researcher who noticed that negative ions had an effect on living things. There were many scientists and researchers who recognized that air electricity (containing both positive and negative charges) stimulates extraordinary growth in plants.

The Italian physicist and Professor Giuseppe Toaldo recognized that plants growing next to a lightning rod grew to ten times the height of identical plants that were just a few feet away.

Jean Antoine Nollet, a French physicist, planted hundreds of mustard seeds in two containers. He electrified one of the containers, using an electrostatic generator.

After a few days, every seed in the electrified container had sprouted and grown a few millimeters, while the seeds in the other container had progressed much more slowly.

Benjamin Franklin's friend, Abbe Bertholon, recognized that when he watered vegetables with a watering can that was electrified by an electrostatic generator, the plants grew to a remarkable size. He spent time creating an 'electrovegetometer' to collect atmospheric electricity by means of an antenna to pass the goodness onto his plants.

Air electricity has been researched by scientists throughout the world and the benefits of air ionization, the process of artificially electrifying the air, has been known to scientists for decades. So much information has been collected, and yet so little has been done with this knowledge. The possibilities for health and disease control provided by nature through air electricity has not yet been fully cultivated.

We are electric

The first book of the Bible, Genesis, describes God as being extremely pleased with the environment that he had created before He put man on the Earth. It then describes the creation of man:

"And the Lord God formed man of the dust of the ground, and breathed into his nostrils the breath of life; and the man became a living soul."

Hindus call breath *prana*. The Chinese call it *chi*, which also means energy. The Taoists view *chi* as having nutritional value and it is sometimes referred to as the "life force".

Ancient textbooks on yoga suggest that a student wishing to perfect his body and mind through breathing exercises should practice near a waterfall, in a cave or, best of all, in a cave under a waterfall. The yoga gurus may not have known about negative ions, but they were familiar with their beneficial effects.

Some Native American tribes understood the healing powers of the air near waterfalls, placing their sick beside a fall to assist with recovery. Similarly, Tai Chi Quan instructors, martial arts *shifu*, Qigong masters and meditation masters advocate deep abdominal breathing in natural settings to promote healing. Eastern healing masters have long recognized this essential element of air, and have developed the art of deep, rhythmic breathing to promote health and longevity.

It is not simply clean air and exercise that makes one feels calm and promotes a good night's sleep. Fresh, unpolluted air is alive with negative ions, which are inhaled, to enter the bloodstream via the lungs, lifting flagging spirits and restoring nature's balance within us.

You might wonder how minute changes in electrical flow could affect your health. But our bodies do not merely produce chemicals. Every healthy cell carries a negative charge, and brain function, in particular, relies as much on correct electrical signals as it does on chemical transfers.

Negative ions help to conduct this vital electric current through the body to ensure optimal cellular functioning.

So the "power grid" in your body is not just an important health factor, but is vital to existence. It has been discovered that rogue cells, such as cancer cells, have a far lower "negative potential" and that somehow causes them to multiply and kill.

Even though science does not recognize such concepts as *chi* or *prana*, modern medicine does not dispute that we are bioelectric beings and life is detected by its electrical activity. In hospitals, bio-electrical technologies such as electrocardiography and electroencephalography are used in medical tests to evaluate the health of the heart and brain.

The claim that something invisible and existing only in the subatomic level is vital to our existence may seem like an old wives' tale or quackery. However, scientists have pointed out that mammals are bioelectric creatures designed by nature to function properly in an environment that contains a certain amount of air electricity. Former NASA scientist James B Beal even wrote that the human race was developed in ionized air.

Kirlian photography, a technique developed in the USSR, strongly supports the theory that the health of all living things must be affected by the different forms of air electricity. This technique, invented in the 1930s by Russian scientist Semyon Kirlian, captures an image of a subject on a sensitized plate when it is exposed to a high electrical voltage on the plate.

The image is a photograph of the strength of the bioelectrical energy, or "aura" of the subject. Photographs of picked leaves taken hours apart show the steady diminishing of bioelectricity as they die. When the technique is applied to sick humans, the aura appears to fade as the bioelectrical energy available diminishes. One supposed benefit of this technique is early diagnosis of serious illnesses like heart disease and cancer.

There are ions in the air around us all the time, but changes in their concentration or in the ratio of positively to negatively charged molecules can have marked biological effects on plants and animals.

A Russian scientist group, headed by ion-science pioneer A.L. Tchijewsky, discovered in 1933 that all animals need ions in the air to live. In an experiment conducted in the USSR, many small animals such as rabbits, guinea pigs, rats, and mice were kept in a well oxygenated atmosphere without any ions present in the air.

All the animals died within 2 weeks from conditions including kidney failure, heart degeneration and fatty liver as a result of the animals' inability to absorb and utilize oxygen. Tchijewsky reported that "an organism receiving the cleanest type of air is condemned to serious illness if the air does not contain at least a small quantity of air ions."

This study strongly suggests that the mere presence of oxygen is not enough to sustain the lives of animals and humans. Air ions are required for the uptake of oxygen into biological bodies for necessary metabolic processes. There have also been similar experiments on plants that resulted in weak and stunted growth. Both positive and negative ions expedite the absorption of iron necessary for the production of plant enzymes.

Additionally, there is much anecdotal evidence of the amazing curative properties of air rich in negative air ions. Many testify to overcoming daunting health challenges simply by going back to nature and breathing nature's fresh, electrified air.

Ion Pioneer Cecil Alfred Laws

Perhaps the first effective home ionizer was developed by Cecil Alfred Laws, one of the outstanding British electronics and radar engineers of the Second World War. He was better known as "Coppy" Laws, a nickname coined by a beautiful and perky young colleague, Rita Hay, who later became his wife.

The sudden death of his father had 14-year old Cecil put up at his school friend's house where he immersed himself in radio, his childhood hobby. He built and installed the first television in the streets where neighbors would gather to watch an hour of weekly BBC broadcasting.

Working by day and attending evening classes by night, sheer determination won him a first class City and Guilds examination in radio communications. Those difficult early years developed in him that persistence and stamina which sustained him throughout his life.

At the breakout of war, Laws was appointed to work on the development of radar. In his twenties, he designed the range finding system that allowed gun to home in on enemy ships with devastating accuracy. The system was first used in March 1941 at the battle of Cape Matapan where the whole Italian fleet was sunk.

Laws also contributed to the development of a radar system that was so accurate in detecting U-boats, submersible warships invented by the Germans, it was instrumental in turning the tide of the war. It was later found that the interiors of the U-boats were ionized, enabling German submarine force to stay underwater for extended period of time. That was perhaps the beginning of Law's fascination with air ionization.

At the age of 51, Laws left a commercially successful career to form his own business and to pursue his interest in ionization. Funding his own research, Laws developed his first ionizer and became an internationally renowned expert in electro-medical science. His company Medion, was later known as Air Ion Technologies and was run by his own son, Julian Laws. Air Ion Technologies carried on research on the use of ionization for the treatment of sick-building syndrome associated with modern buildings and the control of hospital "superbugs". It was eventually dissolved when the director resigned from office.

CHAPTER 2

How the Weather Can Make Us Sick and Stressed

"Those hot dry winds that come down through the mountain passes
and curl your hair and make your nerves jump and your skin itch.
On nights like that every booze party ends in a fight. Meek little wives
feel the edge of the carving knife and study their husband's necks.
Anything can happen"
—Raymond Chandler in Red Wind

My mother was a human weather vane. Whenever her arthritic knee seemed extra troublesome, she would announce with certainty that it was going to rain. "I can feel it in my bones." And she was usually right. How many times have you heard people blaming the weather for their scratchy throat, their aches and pains and general poor health? Whenever there is a drastic change in the weather, complaints of illness abound.

I grew up in a place that is largely populated by descendants of immigrants from neighboring Asian countries. In spite of our cultural and language differences we all share the same prejudices against the weather. "Bad weather" is typically the reason why our children fall sick and even why we have an exceptionally bad day at work.

This kind of folk wisdom does actually have a scientific explanation, however, and it has to do with the electricity of the air.

Biometeorology is the study of how the daily and seasonal weather changes affect animals and humans. While weather influences us all in some way or other, biometeorologists estimate that one in three people are extremely sensitive to weather changes and they may exhibit symptoms associated with atmospheric imbalances due to changing weather.

These symptoms can include migraine headaches, back pain, upset stomach, irritability, loss of appetite, severe depression, feelings of uneasiness, respiratory ills, susceptibility to colds and flu and even hyperactivity. We are not referring here to extremes of heat or cold, but simply to when one atmospheric front gives way to another. At such times of change, weather-sensitive people become extremely miserable. In fact, weather-sensitive people are so affected that they often can predict a weather change, just as my mother did.

How does the weather affect us?

As early as the 19th Century, scientists had found that electricity in the air comes from charged molecules of gas called ions. Changing weather brings about a change in the air ion content and the balance of positive to negative ions in the atmosphere.

While both positive and negative ions are vital to life, an overwhelming number of scientific documents conclude that an overdose of positive ions is harmful, while an overload of negative ions is beneficial.

Nature can bring about an overproduction of positive ions which are generated by friction between air masses, between the wind and the ground, or between weather fronts.

Winds of ill repute

In many parts of the world, seasonal dry winds that sweep across huge expanses of arid landscape bring with them an excess of positive air ions and a myriad of physical and mental ills. The lack of moisture in the air prevents the accumulated positive ions from being conducted to the earth resulting in great electrical disturbances.

In a number of western languages these winds are referred to as the Witches' Winds. Common examples of such winds include the:

- Santa Ana Winds in California
- Mistral in Provence, France
- Northerly Wind in Australia
- Chinook in Canada
- Fonhe in Switzerland & Germany
- Sharav in Israel
- Hamsin in Egypt

"In places where mountains are situated to the south, the south winds that blow are parching and unhealthy; where the mountains are situated in the north, their northern winds occasion disorders and sickness... The winds which must pass over mountains to reach cities do not only dry, but also disturb the air which we breathe and the bodies of men, so as to engender diseases."

Hippocrates, Regimen II, Chapters 37-38

Back in the year 400 BC, Hippocrates, often considered the father of modern medicine, noted that weather has an effect on how well people feel.

Doctors say the Chinook of Canada coincides with outbreaks of the common cold and other respiratory troubles.

Victims of the Swiss Fonhe complain of colds, fatigue, troubled stomachs, depression, sleeplessness, irritability and diminished sex drive. In all these areas, the number of fights, attempted suicides and traffic accidents soar when the 'Witches' Winds' blow.

In the same way, hours or even days before a storm, massive electrical distortions cause a build-up of positive air ions. Weather-sensitive people are the first to react to the imbalanced electricity in the air and to experience inexplicable panic attacks, depression, and irritability, with susceptibility to physical diseases.

It is really more accurate to term these people ion-sensitive rather than weather-sensitive.

It is not just the weather that affects their moods and wellbeing, but the distorted air electricity due to changing weather conditions.

Increased exposure to bad air in winter

During the winter months, the lack of sunshine and green leaves reduces the natural generation of negative ions. Coupled with the need to stay indoors for extended periods, increased amounts of positive ions from sources such as central heating systems, computer devices and electronic appliances continue to bombard our bodies.

Through these months, we languish in ill-ventilated enclosures where positive ions dominate and nature's balance is lost. We become lethargic and slump into illnesses and depression. Seasonal Affective Disorder (SAD) is a form of depression that has been shown to increase in the winter/darker months. Mortality rates in the winter months increase, with cardiac arrests, strokes, pneumonia etc.

American researchers, from the Good Samaritan Hospital in Los Angeles, studied four years of death certificate data from seven states with different winter climates: California, Texas, Arizona, Georgia, Washington, Pennsylvania and Massachusetts. They found that total deaths including cardiac and stroke-related deaths increased by an average of 26 to 36 percent during the winter compared to the summer. Death rates were similar in the winter months throughout the seven states regardless of the temperature.

Early research on negative ionization

Positive ions elevate blood serotonin

Professor Dr Albert Krueger, Emeritus Lecturer in Medicine at the University of California was a microbiologist and renowned ion-scientist. His early work with laboratory mice found that an overdose of positive ions elevates the amount of the hormone serotonin in the blood. An overdose of negative ions, however, had a normalizing effect on blood serotonin.

Serotonin is a neurotransmitter and plays a vital role in regulating mood and general well-being. Changes in blood levels of serotonin can profoundly affect the endocrine glands and central nervous systems. Too much of it has been shown to reduce our ability to function optimally.

Having accumulated a great amount of evidence from his own work and the work of contemporary researchers elsewhere, Dr Krueger postulated that negative air ions stimulate the action of the enzyme monamine oxidase, which is known to metabolize excess serotonin in the body.

On the other hand, positive ions have the opposite effect. They inhibit the effective removal of excessive serotonin from the body. In other words, breathing air rich in negative ions will result in the normalization of blood level serotonin with corresponding beneficial physiological effects.

Dr Felix Sulman was a well-known scientist in the field of biometeorology based at the Hebrew University in Jerusalem. He ran extensive research on the effects of positive and negative ions on human beings. He recognized that positive ions can make people feel bad tempered and irritable but that exposure to negative ions left people feeling more alert, relaxed and happier. Dr Sulman's extensive research also found that too many positive ions can affect the functioning of the thyroid gland.

Dr Sulman first became involved in the study of the effects of exposure to too many positive ions almost by accident. A student doctor invited Dr Sulman to join him in a study of how serotonin was produced by the body and how it affected pregnancy.

Serotonin was first identified in the 1950s as a natural hormone produced when the human body feels under threat or under emotional strain. The production of too much serotonin can be highly detrimental to the wellbeing of humans. Not only can it cause people to suffer depression and heart disease, but it can cause pregnant women to miscarry.

Dr Sulman conducted an experiment to analyze the body's production of serotonin during the time of the Sharav Winds.

These scorching hot, very dry and powerful winds blow for up to 50 days of the year from the desert. Dr Sulman wanted to find the reasons for the ill-effects the Sharav had on the human body.

He invited people who were affected by the Sharav to take part in a medical research study. The urine samples of 200 weather-sensitive people were taken every day and measured for serotonin. It was discovered that during the Sharav their bodies produced up to 1000 percent more serotonin than in times when the wind was not blowing.

Dr Sulman believed that so much serotonin was being produced that people were being poisoned by it.

He identified the effects of serotonin overproduction as migraine headaches, heart pains, breathing difficulties, insomnia, hot flushes, allergic reactions, intestinal spasms, throat infections, irritability, tension and anxiety.

Dr Sulman also suggested that everyone, even normal healthy people, was affected to some extent by atmospheric ion imbalances. While weather-sensitive people overproduce serotonin, the bodies of healthy people typically manufacture adrenaline and noradrenaline, (also known as the 'fight or flight' hormones), in response to these environmental stresses.

Exposure to distorted electricity for a prolonged period of time can therefore lead to great exhaustion. Positive ions may also result in over production of histamine, which makes allergies worse.

Dr Sulman and his team made several interesting discoveries about the effects of the atmospheric ion imbalance caused by the Sharav. Shoe shop sales increased by 300 percent at the time of the winds, as people's feet swelled so much that they had to purchase new footwear. Traffic accidents soared by 100 percent and there was a worsening in the condition of psychiatric patients.

Changes in serotonin production in the body affect the weakest part of the body first. Thus a person with a weak knee (like my mother) may feel the onset of arthritic pains in the knee area when positive ions dominate the air. A veteran with an old war wound may feel the effect of air ion imbalance in the area of the wound. Anyone with a troubling medical condition may experience a worsening of the condition.

"It is the weather," we often hear. Air electricity imbalance is the reason for feeling "under the weather".

The judges take a lenient view

In the nearby Arab countries, the Sharav wind is also known as the Hamsin or the Khamsin. This word means 'fifty' and it refers to the number of days that the wind blows between spring and autumn. The Sharav is also mentioned in the Bible where it is known as the East Wind.

Judges in these countries are known to take a lenient view on violent and aggressive crimes committed during the time that the winds blow. Judges in Switzerland, when the Froehn wind blows, often sentence offenders to a softer punishment than they may have received at another time of the year.

The dangers of man-made weather

We can see from this chapter that people are not actually sensitive to the weather but to the excessive positive charge in the air as a result of changing weather conditions. Fortunately, the natural phenomena that produce positive air ions are transitory. The ill wind does not blow continuously, nor do storms always loom on the horizon.

However, we should be very concerned about the artificial, man-made weather that we have unknowingly created in our homes and offices, in hermetically sealed modern buildings, with central air conditioning.

The modern environment is perpetually charged with positive air ions and sapped of negative ions. This may shed some light as to why many of us struggle with chronic health challenges and never seem to be able to experience any breakthrough.

The unfavorable electrical conditions in which we live and work daily put our body in constant stress. These conditions are just not conducive to our physical and mental healing. Unfortunately, we learn to cope with our pain and discomforts and shortchange ourselves on a vibrant and joy-filled life.

It is important to consider that many problems confronting us every day, such as respiratory ailments, stress-related illness and sleep disorders can be brought about by a lack of negative ions and an overdose of positive ions.

Could the root cause of many of the discomforts relating to the "Sick Building Syndrome" have something to do with ion imbalance in the air inside our homes and office buildings? If so, is there a way to reverse the conditions and create fair weather sanctuaries for us and our families?

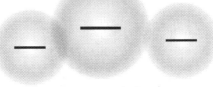

CHAPTER 3

Sick Building Syndrome: How to Create a Healthy Indoor Environment

"God gave His creatures light and air and water open to the skies;
Man locks himself in a stifling lair and wonders why his brother dies."
—Oliver W.Holmes

In spite of the piped music, morale in the computerized data processing room of a South African Bank was low, and many staff took regular sick leave. They complained of headaches, irritability and grumpiness, which carried over after work into their home life. Following the installation of several negative ion generators, the absentee rate went down, the turnover rate normalized and everyone was generally cheerful.

Shortly after the Rothschild Bank of Paris moved into their new modernistic office building, staff began to complain of lethargy, depression, tension, moodiness and feeling below par all the time. Colds and sniffles became common place. A backroom department opted to return to their previous well-ventilated brick office where they had worked for many years and the complaints in that department stopped.

Apparently, the man-made environment of our modern world has taken a toll on inhabitants of cities sprawled across the Earth. Unless a healthy electrical balance is restored to the atmosphere of confined living and working places, the dead, stale air that we breathe consistently on a daily basis will only breed disease and despair.

The environments that we live in today can cause ill health

The highest concentrations of negative ions emanate from natural environments, where nature's balance is unaffected by the hand of man. The reason that we feel lethargic, tired and sluggish or suffer from breathing issues such as hay fever or asthma is that man has altered nature's balance and modern living is not conducive to feeling on top of the world.

Dr L.H. Hawkins, Lecturer in Human Biology and Health at the University of Surrey, UK, collated data on ion concentrations in various locations on fine weather days using a 'Medion" air ion analyzer and his findings are summarized in the following table:

	Air ions/cubic centimeter (cc)	
	Positive Mean (range)	Negative Mean (range)
Outdoors: Clean rural air	1200 (50-2000)	1000 (50-2000)
Outdoors: Lightly polluted urban air	800 (25-1800)	700 (25-1800)
Outdoors: City Air	500 (25-950)	300 (25-750)
Indoors: Rural location, domestic house without air conditioning	1000 (150-1800)	800 (100-1600)
Indoors: Rural location, modern air conditioned office	100 (0-550)	100 (0-400)
Indoor: City location, modern air conditioned office	150 (0-400)	50 (0-400)

Dr Hawkins found that ions quantities are drastically reduced by atmospheric pollution in city areas and further reduced by static electricity or air conditioned systems inside buildings.

Pollution eats up negative ions

In cities, most of the ground is covered by concrete and asphalt, inhibiting the ionizing action of the Earth's surface. Natural Ionization happens all the time, but in the cities, this process is hampered.

Moreover, pollution, caused by the emissions from factories and motor vehicles, reduces the ion count of the urban air. Negative ions are short-lived and readily attach themselves to particles of dust and pollution, conveying a charge to these particles and causing them to clump together and fall to the ground. This clustering behavior of air ions around pollutants result in the formation of large ion clusters which are heavy, sluggish and biologically inactive. Correspondingly, the amount of small negative ions is drastically reduced.

When scientists took measurement of ion count at main intersections of major cities, they detected an average of 50-200 small ions per cubic centimeters at mid-day. In comparison, there are about 2000 to 3000 small ions per cubic centimeter in clean country air.

An electrical engineer commissioned to measure ionization found zero ions during the morning and evening rush hour traffic on a particular freeway in San Francisco. In an atmosphere depleted of negative ions, particles simply drift about on the prevailing air currents, skyrocketing incidences of allergies and breathing problems amongst commuters.

Indoor air can be deadlier than outdoor air

According to the US Environmental Protection Agency, the air inside people's homes can be two to five times more polluted than the air found outside. This is based on the fact that chemical pollutants from all kinds of products we use in our homes and on our bodies accumulate within the ill-ventilated indoor environment, with easily discernible toxic effects.

Recently however, much consideration has also been given to what has been called the electroclimate of the environment and its effects on people. This includes static electric fields, pulsating electric fields, electromagnetic fields and air ions. The theory is that since our body's internal communicative system is brought about by electrical impulses, then external electrical fields will induce stray electrical currents into the system causing subtle but definite disruption to its function.

According to Dr Sydney A. Baggs, PhD, (world authority on heat physics psychology, environmental impact and landscape architecture of earth sheltered architecture), external electromagnetic energy can disturb the biological cycles in the cells of living things, changing the time it takes muscles to react, as well as altering blood chemistry. The immune system is suppressed and diseases such as cancers can result.

Serotonin Irritation Syndrome (SIS)

A condition known as Serotonin Irritation Syndrome, which was first identified as a reaction to overdoses of Serotonin in drug form, has now been identified as being caused mainly by poor indoor air quality with a preponderance of positive air ions.

Professor Albert P. Kreuger of California US was the first to explain the direct effects of excessive positive air ions in causing sudden excessive release of serotonin, a highly active neurochemical, into the bloodstream. The individual's response to an overproduction of serotonin is a range of unpleasant symptoms including migraine, asthma, breathing difficulties, slow thinking, and sensitivity to pain, moodiness, dull-wittedness, sleepiness and emotional irritability.

SIS is triggered by an excessive number of positive charges in the atmosphere exceeding the normal 5 to 4 positive to negative ions ratio.

Unfortunately, this ion imbalance is now characteristic of modern homes and offices and even schools and public institutions. Understanding the environmental factors that cause the effects of SIS is crucial in eliminating indoor pollution and creating a safe and healthy indoor environment.

Air conditioning strips air of negative ions

Our efforts to control our environments have led to the development of artificial means to regulate the indoor climate of our homes, schools, clubs, shops and workplaces.

However, optimizing temperature and humidity in the indoor environment does not necessarily result in an atmosphere that is healthy to the occupants. Despite effective control of temperature, air movement and humidity, a proportion of individuals will complain of lethargy, sleepiness, nausea, or headaches, which they attribute to being in that environment.

In buildings, air conditioning forces the already ion-depleted air from outside through narrow ducts, setting up friction that destroys negative ions leaving positive ions in their place. The design and material of the duct work and the distance the air has to travel to reach the location of the room also determine the amount of positive ions in the air.

Air that comes out of the vents from ducted ventilation systems will have a much greater proportion of positive ions than negative ions. This is further aggravated by the recirculation of air through the ducting. It is thus not unusual to find total depletion of negative ions in a centrally air conditioned room.

Airborne positive charges deplete negative ions

All harmful airborne particles that adversely affect human health such as dust, chemical pollutants, smoke, viruses, bacteria and fungus spores are positively charged. In an environment lacking in negative ions, they stay afloat and diffuse to all available airspace. If the interior is rife with positive ions from the extensive use of synthetic materials, these airborne positive charges will be repelled from surfaces and will continue to circulate in the air that we breathe.

In addition, all forms of combustion like burning, smoking and even breathing take in negative ions and give off positive ones. That is why an ill-ventilated room with an open fire, or people confined in an enclosed space for a prolonged period of time, or a smoke-filled bar, can make one feel suffocated, dizzy or out of sorts.

Static positive charges buildup on synthetic materials

Once in the room, the ions are influenced by airborne dust particles and static surface charges on furniture, fabrics and equipment.

The ceiling, walls and floors of most indoor environments also amass a great volume of positive electrical charges due to the friction of ambient air currents. As these surfaces are rarely made of electrically conductive materials, the buildup of positive charges can be astronomical.

Unless negative ions are replenished continuously through free circulation of fresh outside air or a medical-grade, therapeutic negative air ionizer, these constantly-forming positive charges can deplete the air space of small negative ions, leaving an excess of airborne positive ions.

The widespread use of synthetic materials for our drapes, curtains, carpets and clothes also contributes to an unhealthy indoor environment as friction on synthetic fibers tends to generate positive charges and positive ions. Simply walking across a nylon carpet or wearing a shirt made of synthetic material will produce positive ions.

Try pulling a polyester shirt over your head on a dry day, and you will notice it clings to your body. A lack of moisture in the air inhibits the discharge of these charges to the Earth and static positive charges are built up.

If our clothing has an active positive charge of electricity, then air borne negative ions will be drawn to the clothing, diminishing the number of negative ions available for inhalation. Natural fabrics like cotton and wool do not generate a static charge.

Positively charged, electrostatic fields may be present where large areas of synthetic materials such as carpets, furnishings and building surfaces exist. During dry weather, these surfaces may accumulate up to 100 000 Volts per meter and cause distortion in the body's bioelectric field, which is measured in milliVolts, that is, in thousandths of a Volt.

Christian Bach, a Danish electrical engineer and a pioneer in ion science (*Ions for Breathing* 1967) told of his work as Director in the then Danish Air Ionization Institute and his dealings with a woman who had asthma in her own apartment but not in the apartment of her friend.

Upon investigation, he learnt that most of her furnishings were made from modern synthetic fabrics and her furniture was treated with cellulose or silicon-based furniture finishes which tend to generate a positive charge when rubbed with a polishing cloth.

The furniture of her friend was found to be polished with natural old fashioned wax and elbow grease.

Her asthma attack ceased when her furniture was coated with a natural anti-static compound. She was also told to buy only antique furniture without modern wood treatment.

Mr Bach also quoted another case where one of two enormous henhouses of a chicken farmer experienced an exceptionally high mortality rate. The first henhouse had a roof that was lined with plastic sheets while the other had a wooden roof. A change in wind and weather conditions affected the air electricity and caused the plastic to overproduce positive ions causing the demise of a great number of chickens.

Unnatural materials will cause an imbalance of air ions which may result in a range of nagging symptoms and aggravation of respiratory problems. Asthmatics and allergy suffers will find that they can drastically improve their breathing space by using only things made from natural materials.

Earthing That Positive Charge

Recently, there has been great interest in the health benefits of earthing or "nature contact". Walking bare feet on the Earth's natural surfaces such as grass, sand, or dirt, digging one's hands into the soil during gardening, as well as contact with trees and shrubs, are said to make for relaxation and good health.

What happens when we contact the earth? One effect is that we discharge accumulated static charges on our body into the earth.

Our bio-electric body is conductive and free electrons as well as charged ions (called electrolytes) are conveyed within the body via the blood and other body fluids which are good conductors.

If we are insulated from the ground with synthetic or rubber shoes, the flow of positive electric charges to the negatively charged earth is obstructed and a static electrical field can build up on all the surfaces of the body and clothing. Small negative ions around the body are lost through neutralization and we are surrounded by an increasing field density of positive ions. Positive air ions are repelled into the air from these surfaces and we breathe them in.

All this is to the great detriment of human health, performance and comfort. As you will discover in later chapters, inhaling excessive positive ions can suppress the immune system, cause sleeplessness, and greatly undermine our respiratory health and mental well-being, augmenting feelings of tension, anxiety, depression. Static charges on the body have also been linked to skin rash.

"Earthing" cannot happen when we are using synthetic or rubber soled shoes which inhibit the transfer of positive static charges into the earth.

If you have ever run across new-mown grass on a dry, sunny day in rubber soled joggers, you will have noticed that your legs are covered in grass due to an accumulated charge caused by friction between the joggers and the ground.

Carpet made from synthetic materials and ground surfaces of asphalt, wood, vinyl, tar or plastic also cut off our connection to the earth.

To ensure a continual removal of static charges from the body, wear natural leather shoes or go bare feet as often as possible. When you have been trapped inside a modern building full of electropollution, try touching the earth or trees to drain off those destructive charges. You may be surprised with the almost immediate sense of wellbeing.

The pressing need to improve indoor air quality

A typical urban resident spends 90 percent of his/her time indoors, in tightly-sealed air conditioned buildings with most furnishings made from synthetic materials, which generate large volumes of positive ions. Airborne dust particles and chemical molecules from chemical aerosols, detergents and furniture finishes, appliances and paints also continuously deplete the air of negative ions, leaving an excess of positive ions.

Negative ions are also used up by people as they breathe. As a result, humans often live or work in confined spaces where positive ions reign. We can be left feeling exhausted, with a lower immunity against respiratory illnesses, cancers and depression. We feel weak and tired in this type of environment but we are expected to be creative, productive, motivated and feel good.

Sick building syndrome (mentioned in detail above) is an example of how a lack of negative ions can fill workers with malaise. In the airtight enclosure typical of a modern office, there is serious ion depletion resulting in allergic reaction, lethargy and disease germs incubating and passing from one person to another.

Indicators identified by the World Health Organization as being common symptoms of Sick Building Syndrome include:

- Breathing difficulties or wheeziness
- Sore throat
- Dry throat
- Cold or flu like symptoms
- Rashes or itches
- Tiredness or fatigue
- Blocked or running nose
- Dry itchy and tired eyes
- Coughs and/or sneezes
- Headaches
- Sleeping difficulties
- Short term memory
- Concentration problems
- Depression/pessimism
- Irritability/tension

In offices, there is loss of productivity and man-hours due to absenteeism caused by bad indoor air quality.No wonder the American Lung Association and the EPA identified indoor air quality as one of the top five most urgent environmental risks to public health.

Unfortunately, city dwellers are working and living in unnatural environments with greatly distorted air electricity for the greater part of their lives. Additionally, they travel in closed motor vehicles, shop in malls with a delicately engineered climate and work out in indoor gymnasiums where body conscious individuals are packed together sweating and breathing second hand air.

We have unknowingly put ourselves at risk of both physical and mental problems by subjecting ourselves to a chronic environmental stress that exerts pressure on our body chemistry.

How to create a healthy indoor environment

Step 1) Ventilate, ventilate, ventilate

The ancient Chinese knew that life lies in motion. "Flowing water never stagnates, and the hinges of an active door never rust." Here, Confucius was referring to the importance of movement, for when movement ceases, energy stagnates. In the same way, air trapped within our modern air-tight apartments becomes sluggish and heavy with accumulating positive ions. People breathing in the dead air become sleepy, dull-witted and irritable.

In medieval England, houses that were not located in positions that allowed the continuous renewal of air by breezes were considered bad houses. The early craftsmen were to be mindful to structure houses that gave admission to winds for when the air stagnates, contagion ensues.

We have seen above how occupants of buildings that do not contain fresh air suffer. They complain of symptoms such as headaches, eye, nose and throat irritation, fatigue, dizziness and nausea. They also report itchy skin and difficulty with concentrating. Complainants report that as soon as they leave the building, they feel better. These symptoms are thought to be brought on by negative-ion starvation and positive ion poisoning within an ill-ventilated room.

The buildup of positive charges in the indoor environment can be neutralized by negative ions through circulation of fresh air outside. People are more willing to open the windows during warmer weather, but in the winter months, we can also leave a window or two open just a crack to allow some fresh air to flow through the home.

An opened window allows healthy negative ions to enliven the room, removing dampness and odors and admitting the sweet scents and sounds of nature's gifts.

Step 2) Keep house plants, build water fountains

The indoor environment has become a health hazard, with every modern fixture and furnishing promoting the generation of positive ions and thwarting the replenishment of healthy negative ions. It follows that we would want our indoor air to be like natural air in its most nurturing form, rich in negative ions.

Waterfalls and tropical forests and crashing waves at the beach produce large amounts of negative ions. It helps explain the good feeling people experience at these places. A walk through a forest is also a Japanese therapy for mental stress called Shinrinyoku.

Notably, as plants emit water vapors through transpiration, they produce negative ions. America's National Aeronautics and Space Agency in partnership with the Association Landscape Contractor of America recommend house plants as a mean to improve air quality.

Dr Lohr from Washington State found that houseplants can reduce human stress, increase productivity, lift moods and cut down dust. This is likely due to the increased number of negative ions produced by the plants. In another study, it was found that placement of houseplants in a computer room reduces dust level by 20 percent, significantly reducing allergies and housekeeping time.

Recognizing the beneficial psychological effects that living plants have on humans, the Japanese are now adding "Ecology Gardens" to Tokyo hospitals. It has been observed that when plants are present, patients in hospital experience shorter recovery times.

The energy of falling water frees electrons from neutral particles of air, adding to the proportion of negative ions. Architects and designers are beginning to appreciate the wisdom of the ancient Roman culture and to realize the health benefits of fountains and rooftop solariums placed in urban environments. Waterfall spas, known for their therapeutic effects, are also gaining widespread popularity amongst the healthy conscious.

In some cultures falling water fountains are considered to be a necessary part of a healthy indoor landscape. Feng Shui is the ancient Chinese art of placement and arrangement of space to achieve harmony with the environment. This ancient Chinese practice is still being employed to promote a healthy living environment. Water fountains, sprays and ferns are some of the chief items used to achieve harmony, health and wellness. All these items generate negative ions and improve air quality.

The shower in our homes is also a built-in, natural ionizer. This mini man-made waterfall produces negative ions making our daily bath rituals such refreshing, vitalizing and enjoyable experiences.

Step 3) Eliminate the causes of indoor pollutants

Almost all the objects that we use as part of our everyday lives shed particles or give off onerous gases. This is particularly true when articles are new. Clothing, curtains, carpets, and other fibers are shed into the air that we breathe. In our pursuit of cleanliness, we use liquid and aerosol detergents to clean furniture, floors and dishes. Of the hundreds of toxic chemicals found indoors, a large number of these chemicals have the potential to cause not only allergic reactions, but also cancer and other forms of illness.

While daily housekeeping can and does remove some of the larger harmful particles, many smaller ones still circulate in the air and are inhaled by us. These pollutants are very light, being less than 1 micron in size, and they include potentially dangerous bacteria, viruses, fungi spores and gaseous molecules of volatile organic compounds (VOC). Some common examples of hazardous VOCs found in the home are benzene, formaldehyde and trichloroethylene. In our airtight energy-efficient homes and offices where there is a lack of natural air ions, these small particles may never settle but remain airborne.

We can clean up our indoor air by:

- constantly replenishing the negative air ions through ventilation or other means;
- reducing the use of household chemicals and switching to cleaning products and paints that do not contain VOCs. Baking soda, vinegar and borax are effective natural cleaning alternatives;
- airing dry-cleaned clothes outdoor before bringing them into the house;
- using and buying only small quantities of chemical products to eliminate the need to store such items in the house.

Step 4) Install a negative air ionizer

A therapeutic, medical-grade negative air ionizer has become a modern necessity. The atmosphere of our modern homes and offices is depleted in health-giving negative air ions. Often it is not practical to open the window for free circulation of fresh air because of acute outdoor pollution. In many large corporate offices, it is not even possible to open the windows to allow fresh air to enter the building.

Electrically generating the necessary negative ions and propagating them continuously throughout the closed environment with a negative air ionizer is an effective and economic solution.

In fact, occupational health experts recommend air ionization as an extremely cost-effective means of enhancing health and productivity in indoor workplaces.

The abundance of negative ions produced by an ionizer negates the effect of the accumulation of static positive charges on interior surfaces. Airborne positive ions as well as positively charged particles of dust, germs, and chemical gas molecules also attract negative ions which convey a charge to the particles. The charged particles then cluster together and fall to the ground, settling as visible dust on surfaces.

Germs and harmful microbes are similarly charged and destroyed leaving a clean bacteria-free atmosphere where we can safely spend our working and leisure hours.

The value of ionizing the indoor atmosphere of the workplace is demonstrated in a collaborative work by John Jukes of WESTRA (Workplace Environment Science & Technology Research Assoc) and representatives from British Telecoms and Air Ion Technologies. The researchers studied the effects of air ionization on the health and productivity of 1159 office, control room and call-center staff, in eight different locations over a six-year period.

During the trial, an elaborate symptom scoring system was used with extensive direct interviews to quantify the extent of improvement in human health and performance due to the artificial generation of negative ions in modern working environments via air ionizers. Despite a variety of building structures, interior furnishing, air ventilation systems, and types of activity, the studies showed a surprising consistency of before and after symptom patterns.

There was an average 57.9% improvement in all 10 indicators of Sick Building Syndrome due to ionization, with a significant 71% reduction in headaches. The ionizers also contributed to 38% reduction in general stress symptoms and a 35% reduction in sickness absence.

The researchers concluded that ionization of the ambient air in the workplace brought about substantial reductions in sickness symptoms and sickness absenteeism with significant improvements in productivity.

Environmental Stress	Due to Ionisation		
	Before	After	%Impr
Breathing difficulties	275.3	90.6	67.1
Sore throat	474.3	197.9	58.3
Dry Throat	834.4	497.2	40.4
Cold/Flu like symptoms	681.9	270.4	60.3
Rashes or itches	437.8	285.8	34.7
Tiredness/ fatigue	1019.5	495.0	66.0
Blocked or runny nose	740.5	324.5	56.2
Dry, itchy, tired eyes	863.4	330.6	73.2
Cough/sneezing	808.6	391.8	51.6
Headaches	745.0	302.6	71.6
Average improvement			57.9%

General Stress	Part due to ionization		
	Before	After	%impr
Sleeping difficulties	581.8	390.3	32.9
Short term memory	427.1	285.0	33.3
Concentration problems	697.5	383.0	37.0
Depressed/ pessimistic	482.0	268.6	44.3
Irritable tense	904.2	529.2	41.5
Average improvement			38%

Tabulated results from the study of the *Impact of Improved Air Quality on Productivity and Health in the Workplace* conducted by John Jukes, Andrew Jenkins and Julian Laws.

Bankers in South Africa also reported an 80% reduction in data entry error rate after the installation of air ionizers in their offices.

Professor A P Krueger reported on a Swiss bank of over 600 employees: for every one day lost among the group of people working in negative ion enriched air, there were sixteen lost among the people working in normal air.

Dr Hawkins at Surrey University also noted that negative ions provided up to 29% improvement in the ability of his students to perform high concentration psycho-motor tasks over performing the same tests in normal indoor conditions.

Choosing an air ionizer

In choosing an air ionizer, we should beware of the extravagant claims of manufacturers of inferior ionizing machines. Many of these machines lose their effectiveness over time or generate potentially harmful by-products of ozone and other oxides that can be detrimental to the health if breathed in over a prolonged period of time.

The Himalayan salt crystal lamp has also been marketed as a natural air ionizer. However, the truth is that Himalayan Salt Crystal lamps do not produce negative ions at all. This can easily be proven with the use of an atmospheric ion analyzer.

Give me any such lamp and my ion analyzer will register zero ion count. Any health effects from these lamps come from their dehumidifying capabilities. Drier air may provide some degree of relief for asthmatics and those with breathing difficulties.

Similarly, many disappointed buyers have failed to receive any benefits from products marketed as ionizers that do not emit ions. (In Chapter 10, you will find the eight things that you should consider when choosing an air ionizer.)

Step 5) Avoid the Use of Synthetics

Synthetics generate positive charges which contribute to an unhealthy indoor environment. Choose clothes and furnishings made from natural materials whenever possible. Facilitate nature contact by wearing shoes that allow accumulated static positive charges to be 'earthed'; or go bare feet as often as possible.

Electrosmog—A new kind of deadly pollution

Electromagnetic fields are present everywhere in our environment even though they are invisible to the human eye. Energy from the Earth's surface not only produces ions, but creates an electrical field as well. The Earth's natural magnetic field causes a compass needle to orient in a North-South direction and is used by birds, insects and fish for navigation.

In the Earth's atmosphere, there are electromagnetic waves of extremely low frequencies. One such frequency is the Schumann Resonance (7.83Hz) which corresponds with the waves of the brain that are known to produce anxiety-relieving and stress-reducing effects. This brain frequency also controls our creativity, performance and immune system.

It is said that all living things on the Earth, including humans, are

> ### Human Brain Wave Frequencies
>
> **Beta waves** *range between 13-40 Hz. The beta state is associated with peak-concentration, heightened alertness and visual acuity*
>
> **Alpha waves** *range between 7-12 Hz. The Alpha state is a place of deep relaxation and meditation. In Alpha, we begin to access the wealth of creativity-that lies just below our conscious awareness*
>
> **Theta waves** *range between 4-7 Hz. Theta is a state of somnolence with reduced consciousness. It has also been-identified as the gateway to learning and memory.*
>
> **Delta waves** *range between 0-4 Hz. Delta is associated with deep sleep with the release of Human Growth Hormone beneficial for healing and regeneration.*
>
> *Adapted from Dr. Aurelie Laurence's blog post "What are the Frequencies of Human Brain Waves?"*

under the influence of the Schumann Resonance to maintain the basic rhythm of life. The Schumann Resonance has also been called the "pulse of life."

The human brain waves range between 0 to 40 Hz. When asleep, our brain activity can be measured at between 0 to 7 Hz; when awake it is between 10 to 15 Hz.

Another characteristic of the brain is that it functions like a tuning fork. It picks up an external electrical influence and alters its brain wave pattern to resonate with that frequency. Thus, variation and distortions in the atmospheric electrical field will have a biological effect on human beings.

Going outside during fair weather helps our brain frequency to attune to the natural oscillation frequency of the atmospheric field, which being the same as our brain's most relaxed yet alert state, enhances our alertness and improves reaction time. This perhaps accounts for the good feeling of being outdoors during fair weather.

Alarmingly, 21st century technologies have saturated the atmosphere with man-made electromagnetic fields that are some ten million times stronger than the average natural background. This is unprecedented and completely unnatural.

EMF Hazards

Electromagnetic fields (EMFs) or electromagnetic radiation (EMR), have become broad terms used to describe energy waves created by the vast array of electrical devices and wireless technologies. EMFs include

- Extremely Low Frequencies (ELF) from electrical appliances, (between 50-60Hz) and
- Radio Frequency radiation (RF) from wireless devices such as mobile phones, cordless phones, laptop computers, WI-FI and WI-MAX networks, and radio transmission networks (between 100,000 Hz to 100 000 000Hz)

These technologies are designed for convenience and energy efficiency, without due consideration of the biological effects on people. For years, prominent scientists have warned of the dangers of EMR as a source of health problems. Hundreds of case histories documenting changes in people's health and quality of life as a result of exposures leave no doubt that such dangers exist.

A signwriter had gradually declined in health and work ability to about 6 hours' work per day and suffered greatly from depression and head noises as well as poor sleep patterns. It was found that he worked in his signwriting workshop with his head always within 25 centimeters of three double 40 watt fluorescent light fittings.

He was advised to replace these fittings with incandescent bulbs, and within three to four weeks of the lights being changed, his health was restored and he could work up to 12 hours a day without any fatigue.

Although fluorescent lights are more efficient than ordinary incandescent bulbs, they require a ballast transformer that generates an ELF field. An incandescent lamp, on the other hand, generates virtually no ELF.

Extensive research also shows that Radio Frequency radiations from mobile phones, phone masts and WIFI significantly reduce the body's production of the hormone melatonin, a sleep regulator and anti-cancer agent. This could result in sleep disorders and increased incidence of cancer. Research also demonstrates that exposure to such radiation destroys the blood-brain barrier, allowing toxins to pass into the brain leading to dizziness, headaches, disorientation and in the long term, brain cell degeneration.

Clusters of cancer and other serious illnesses such as brain hemorrhages and high blood pressure have been discovered around mobile phone masts raising public concerns about the safety of the technology.

One such cluster site is a small village in Cornwall, UK. Within the two years after a mobile mast was erected in Buckler, Cornwall, half of the residents had complained of serious ill health with many experiencing severe headaches, vertigo, depression and lack of sleep

Eight residents had since died from cancer and several more were being diagnosed with the disease.

The World Health Organization (WHO), in response to public and governmental concern, established the International Electromagnetic Fields (EMF) Project in 1996 to assess the scientific evidence of possible adverse health effects from electromagnetic fields. Subsequently in May 2011, the International Agency for Research on Cancer (IARC), a WHO specialized agency, classified radiofrequency electromagnetic fields as possibly carcinogenic to humans.

In 2007, the BioInitiative Working Group released a 650-page report on more than 2,000 studies indicating a definitive link between EMFs and serious health problems.

Chronic exposure can impair immunity, cause a variety of cancers, Alzheimer's disease, dementia, heart disease, autism and many other disorders. Decades of international scientific research confirms that EMFs from all artificial sources have a toxic effect on the human body.

Remember we are electrical beings. Our body's own internal electrical system functions with very weak electrical impulses that are generated by the brain and used for intercellular communication.

Long term exposure to external electric fields, many times stronger than the body's own bioelectrical signals, can disrupt the body's communication system and adversely affect health.

The truth, however, is that for the first time in human history we are surrounding ourselves and our children with an ever-thickening "electrosmog".

Although it is hard to imagine a world without mobile communication and electrical conveniences, our young children are at the highest risk for long-term health problems from this pervasive health threat.

Fortunately, there are easy ways to keep these pollutants at bay. The following are suggestions to help minimize your exposure:

- Avoid using microwave ovens, Bluetooth devices, mobile phones, and cordless phones whenever possible;
- Use incandescent bulbs instead of fluorescent lamps for close-up work or desk lighting;
- Keep a safe distance from wireless devices or turn them off when not in use;
- Use the speakerphone function or wired headset when using a cell phone;
- Use a corded phone if possible;
- Live away from high-power lines or cell phone masts;
- Unplug or turn off all electrical appliances at the power point when not in use; (Turning most devices off at the unit does not turn the power supply off. The power supply continues to operate and the device continues to radiate.)
- If you are concerned about EMF levels in your home or work environment, buy an EMF detector to help you identify hotspots in order to modify them;
- Use energy tools with brain entrainment technologies to align yourself with healing frequencies. Incidentally, medical grade air ionizers frequently incorporate such technologies to produce frequencies that have proven beneficial effects on the human body. They can be configured to pulse negative ions at frequencies to help overcome specific health problems or to induce sleep, dream or other brainwave changes (see Chapter 9 for more detail).

Re-creating fresh indoor air is the first step to restoring our physical and mental equilibrium, as we spend a great part of our lives inside buildings. Fresh air also helps us cope with stress. The advice to "take a breather" in order to relax and unwind has always been welcomed.

One of most obvious common sense stress and anger management tips is to take a deep breath and count to ten. Experts tell us that stress often causes us to breathe shallowly and this in turn almost always causes more stress.

In the next chapter, we will see how balancing air electricity can help us alleviate serious stress symptoms and eliminate stress permanently.

CHAPTER 4

The Intelligent Way to Eliminate Stress

"You can increase the oxygen currents of nerve force with the
breath and send it to heal parts of your body."
—Paul C. Bragg

I n this modern age, it's easy to get stressed. After all, there is so
much that we need to do in order to thrive in the hectic society
that we have created for ourselves. Information is more readily
available and we are constantly battered with marketing messages,
bad news and reasons to be fearful all while we are trying to make a
living and do what we need to do to eat and take care of ourselves.

But stress is not to be taken lightly for it is the underlying cause of
almost all illness and disease. The United States government says in a
research study on the CDC website that stress causes over 90 percent
of sicknesses. Most medical doctors agree that the immune system is
capable of healing anything if it is not suppressed by stress. In other
words, stress not only causes physical illness but also perpetuates it.
The negative emotional states that are associated with having too
much stress are anxiety, depression and anger.

Today's hectic lifestyles

An example of the hectic lifestyle is that of the working mother who has three offspring to be concerned about. Not only does she have to tend to the physical, emotional and educational needs of her children, she also has a house to run and a husband to care for. Her husband is equally busy trying to advance himself on a highly competitive and political career ladder. It is hard to find any time to relax and life can at times be overwhelming and too much to handle.

Let's call our busy housewife, Janice.

Looking for a solution, Janice goes to her doctor who is fairly laid back when it comes to prescribing medication. He suggests that she tries taking sleeping pills for those times that she feels anxious and has trouble sleeping. He might not mention the side effects that she could suffer, such as brain lacerations or respiratory issues, or even that during the night if her children wake and need her, she may not be able to wake up to care for them.

We know that it may not be a good fit for Janice to start taking sleeping pills. There are other solutions to her dilemma. Ion research from around the world demonstrates that breathing air with high negative ion content helps conserve body energy supply and improves respiration thereby increasing overall energy and vitality.

Besides that, negative ions also negate the effects of stress hormones so that one can better cope with a busy lifestyle. Bad air on the other hand, induces stress by causing our bodies to produce bio-chemicals that have psychological side effects. Improving nutrition and correcting deficiencies can also help us with our mental wellbeing.

Distorted air electricity and aggression

Humankind has a knack for creating disharmony in the name of progress. We saw in Chapter 3 how in cities everywhere, in cars, trains, buses, planes, high rise office buildings and apartments, nature's supply of air electricity has been so restricted that most of us find city life extremely exhausting.

We get locked into so called "ion prisons" for hours at a time, exposed to lethal doses of positive ions created by modern technology. Our bodies over secrete serotonin in response to this electrical abnormality, causing symptoms that range from inexplicable anxieties and tension, feelings of weariness or unnatural bursts of hyperactivity to serious psychiatric problems.

In Chapter 2 we read of how dry seasonal winds in some parts of the world bring about imbalances in the natural electrical charge of the air and can cause increased aggression and depression. A 1971 issue of Time magazine reported that the dry ionizing Khamsin wind in Egypt brought about aberrant behavior, with rampant automobile accidents and a 20 percent increase in the crime rate.

Eric Marsden, the distinguished staff correspondent for London Sunday Times in Jerusalem during the seventies, noted increased hostility between Israeli Jews and Arabs along the West Bank during the days of the Sharav (the Israeli equivalent of the Khamsin). Listless soldiers with hair-trigger tempers produced a palpable tension in the air which threatened to erupt in a bloody shambles.

However, these are temporary phenomena unlike the perpetual unhealthy environments we have created for ourselves in our cities. While we may think that our emotional and mental upheavals are due to a stressful job or a domestic rift, it is just as likely that the unhealthy electrical climate is the reason why we find our jobs stressful or fight with our partners at home in the first place.

Bullying has also been attributed to the unhealthy ionic environment in schools and especially in locker rooms, with low ceilings and steel depositories which intensify the amount of positive ions in the air.

Researchers have studied the behavioral effects of air ions through scientific experiments. Laboratory mice and rats were exposed to positive ions and they became aggressive and agitated.

Dr Felix Gad Sulman is known internationally as one of the leaders in negative ion research. We read of his research among weather-sensitive people during the Sharav in Chapter 2.

Dr Sulman discovered that when his subjects were exposed to an overload of positive ions for an hour, they become bad tempered, fatigued and irritable. The same people confined in a room full of negative ions felt much better and were alert and relaxed. Dr Sulman went on to test their alertness and capacity for work and found that they scored significantly higher during and after exposure to negative ions.

Negative ions as mood elevators

Even though we cannot sense them working, negative ions have been found to have a major effect on mood. In fact, positively charged air ions have been termed "grouchy" ions while negatively charged ions, "happy" ions. Improvement in moods has been repeatedly demonstrated in patients exposed to negative ions.

Researchers found that those suffering from Seasonal Affective Disorder (SAD) improved from exposure to negative ions. SAD is a recognized form of depression that is brought on by not having enough exposure to sunshine and is particularly prevalent in the Nordic countries such as Scandinavia.

Dr Michael Terman, Professor of Clinical Psychology at Columbia University in New York, uses negative ion making machines to treat those who suffer from depression and SAD during the wintertime. This therapy has been found to work almost as well as light therapy for the winter blues.

Ionization therapy had already been used experimentally to treat depression. In 1992, Dr Michael J. Norden, a psychiatrist and clinical Associate Professor at the University of Washington purchased a medical grade air ionizer as a possible alternative to treating depressed patients with powerful drugs. He later wrote in his book *Beyond Prozac*: "Ionization therapy shows tremendous potential."

Researchers at Columbia University also discovered that sufferers of chronic depression could relieve symptoms with the use of negative ions. Negative ions metabolize and neutralize serotonin in much the same way as one of the prescribed groups of anti-depressant drugs, known as MAO inhibitors.

MAO inhibitors are reserved as the last line of treatment because of potentially lethal dietary and drug interactions. In contrast, ionization therapy has been found to be a safe, effective alternative without the side effects that can occur with taking a pharmaceutical pill. This safe, drug-free treatment for depression was later patented by the University in July 1996.

In essence, this treatment involves the use of high density negative ions of oxygen for depressive disorders characterized by excessive sleepiness, fatigue and carbohydrate cravings.

Dealing with anxiety

Anxiety is one of the most common afflictions of modern humanity. According to the Anxiety and Depression Association of America, 18 percent of the U.S. population is affected by anxiety disorders. While some degree of anxiety may be beneficial, as it acts as a motivator for change and improvement, many people suffer from the destructive state of chronic anxiety, which is often attributed to the pace of modern life.

Anxiety and depressive disorders are the major causes of chronic insomnia. Anti-anxiety drugs also known as sedatives are often prescribed to reduce feelings of tension and anxiety, and to induce sleep. Anti-anxiety medications are among the most abused drugs in the United States.

All the symptoms of the disorder described as anxiety psychoneurosis are similar to those described by victims of positive ion poisoning. Dr Sulman's Sharav-victim patients complained of insomnia, irrational anxiety, inexplicable depression, unnamed fears, irritability, sudden panic attacks, uncertainty and constant colds. These are caused by drastic bio-chemical changes that occur in the body on prolonged exposure to an electrically imbalanced atmosphere. In effect, the victim's body is poisoned by serotonin produced by their own bodies.

It is interesting to note that almost all cases of anxiety psychoneurosis are presented to doctors, psychiatrists and psychologists in cities and urban areas, where serious ion depletion and positive ion poisoning occur in modern homes and offices. If serotonin over production stimulated by high amounts of atmospheric positive ions causes such mental disorders, then a reversing of symptoms could be brought about by exposure to negative ions which convert excess serotonin into a harmless chemical.

In Romania, a comprehensive study of the benefits of ionization was carried out involving 100 outpatients at a mental health clinic. After five sessions of forty to fifty minutes of exposure to negative air ions, normal sleep returned in 80 percent of insomnia patients. 75 percent of headache patients reported that their pain had disappeared. Over half of depressive patients claimed a return to 'normal', while all anxiety sufferers said their symptoms had disappeared.

Protection against stress and exhaustion

Stress is unique to every individual. What stresses one person may not stress another. Two people in exactly the same situation may have completely different responses.

Psychologist Dr Alexander Loyd N.D., PhD is an expert in energy healing. He explains that the critical element of stress is always internal.

Stress is not caused by something outside us, but our unique internal programming causes us to perceive something as threatening or stressful. While Dr Loyd is referring to the cellular memories of our bodies and our unique life experiences that make us the person that we are, our internal chemical composition will also influence our responses to potentially unsettling events.

Picture two motorists stuck in rush hour traffic; we have all seen how differently people react to this situation. After an hour of bumper to bumper traffic, and being cooped up in the small closed cabin with a totally unnatural ionic atmosphere, the first driver becomes tense, anxious and highly strung. He may even experience road rage. The other driver, having established a healthy micro-climate within his motor vehicle with a negative ion generator, is as cool as a cucumber while going through the same exasperating traffic condition.

Reports from Hungary, Japan, the USA, and Britain support findings that the buildup of positive ions inside vehicles leads to drivers' fatigue and loss of co-ordination. Positive ion overdose inflicted on car drivers also causes them to become tense and liable to lose their tempers. Unhealthy positive ion concentration in cars also accounts for cranky kids and rows between husband and wife, and presents a threat to driver, passengers and other road users.

In coping with stress and indeed all issues of daily life, we need to stack the deck in our favor and do all we can to remain high functioning, productive and self-controlled. If we are highly strung, it would only take a little tiff or a thoughtless word to overload the system and cause a fuse to blow somewhere in the psyche.

Psychiatric medications include antidepressants, stimulants, antipsychotics, mood stabilizers, anxiolytics and depressants, and are designed to exert an effect on the chemical makeup of the brain and nervous system. They are widely used to treat mental disorders, clinical depression, anxieties, hyperactivity and other disorders. Ironically, some of these medications may actually cause the problems that they are supposed to treat.

Recently, there has been concern that the use of antidepressant medications may induce suicidal behavior in youths. In 2004, the U.S. Food and Drug Administration (FDA) issued a public warning about an increased risk of suicidal thoughts or behavior in children and adolescents treated with SSRI antidepressant medications.

Studies into a series of school shootings during an 18 year period from 1988-2006 showed that in most cases, the shooters were either on or withdrawing from these types of psychiatric medication. Just as with abnormal air electricity, a pharmaceutical drug can also exert pressures on our body chemistry and influence us to think and behave in destructive ways.

Malnutrition can also cause depression, anxiety and other mental disorders. Could it be that our modern diet comprising of mainly nutrient-depleted processed foods and convenient fast foods are causing an epidemic of ill health?

A balanced food supply can keep all kinds of diseases at bay. Barbara Stitt, author of *Food & Behavior: A Natural Connection*, was a former probation officer. She found that when ex-offenders changed their diet, they lost their hostility and other symptoms that would cause them to act out in a criminally offensive manner.

Dr. Weston A. Price, a dentist and researcher in the 1930s found that primitive tribes eating a natural whole food diet high in animal foods and animal fats were extremely healthy physically and mentally. They also had strong moral characters and had no need for prisons.

Deficiency in vitamin Bs, such as B1, B2, B6 and B12, can produce fears, hostility, depression, fatigue, confusion, anxiety, rage and paranoia which are also symptoms of neuropsychiatric disorders. For example, Pellagra is an extreme condition of niacin (vitamin B3) deficiency.

People suffering from pellagra not only have skin problems, but also show symptoms of mental illness. According to Dr. Andrew Saul who co-authored the excellent book, *Niacin: The Real Story*, high doses of niacin have been successfully used in the treatment of mental and behavioral disorders, such as attention deficit disorder, general psychosis, anxiety, depression, obsessive-compulsive disorder or bipolar disorder.

If stress is getting you down, why not first correct your air, and your diet? Breathe fresh electrified natural air and eat good food to help balance up those complex internals. Dr Andrew Saul says that two handfuls of cashews will give you the therapeutic equivalent of a prescriptive dose of Prozac. If necessary, consider taking a niacin supplement and consult your physician regarding the effective dosage.

In summary, here are things you can start doing right away to help you eliminate stress for a healthy body and mind:

Step 1) Consistently breathe fresh, ionized air

Breathing good quality air will help tame those nerves, energize your body and give you clarity of mind and focus so that you can apply your brain to solutions.

Step 2) Avoid convenience foods

Ditch those dead de-vitalized processed convenience foods and opt for real foods that will fuel your body and mind. Correct deficiencies and supplement where necessary.

Step 3) Simplify and sort out your priorities

Sometimes it helps to step back and assess if what we have is worth keeping and what we are doing is worth continuing. Get rid of everything in your life you don't absolutely need. The only thing you need is your healthy body, integrity and love. After you have simplified your house and life, you will find your breaths becoming lighter and easier. Unknowingly we have been weighed down with a lot of unnecessary load.

Step 4) Use an energy tool to deal with past trauma

Memories of past traumas can cause a lot of stress and harm to our bodies if not dealt with properly. Instead of suppressing them, neutralize those negative energies with an energy tool. Dr Alexander Loyd and his scientific healing protocol known as *The Healing Codes* are helping many people reverse physical and mental symptoms due to stresses caused by destructive memories.

Step 5) Manage your money matters

According to a recent survey in Britain, nearly three-quarters of adults suffer disturbed nights to due to money worries. Good money management is necessary for peace of mind and general wellbeing. It is important to keep track of how much money you have coming in, and how much you have to set aside for essential bills. Don't be tempted to buy on credit but instead eliminate all debts. Simplify your life.

A spokesperson for British mental health charity Mind, said, "If you are struggling to keep control of your money, you may find that your mental health is affected. Likewise, if you are experiencing a period of mental ill health you may find that you get into financial difficulties." So eliminate all the stress relating to financial matters by managing your resources wisely. FamilyFoundations.com conducts seminars as well as publishes books that teach sound biblical-based financial principles you may wish to check out.

Step 6) Get out into the sunshine

Natural sunshine is a proven cure for depression. Experts have often cited the association between sunlight exposure and mood. A recent study published in Environmental Health found that a lack of sunshine exacerbates cognitive and memory problems in people suffering from depression.

Seasonal Affective Disorder, which often occurs during the long winter months, usually fades in spring as the hours of daylight increase.

Sunlight helps our body to synthesize Vitamin D, which is not only essential for bone health but has also been shown to reduce respiratory infections and other illness. Bare as much of your skin as you dare for appropriate periods and soon you will find that you are feeling much better.

Step 7) Take exercise

According to the Mayo Clinic, besides preventing and improving a number of health problems, physical exercise can also help reduce anxiety and improve mood. In addition to forcing you to breathe in lots of negative ions, especially if you exercise outdoors, meeting exercise goals can boost one's confidence, as can improvement in one's physique and appearance as a result of exercise.

Exercise also provides a temporary distraction from the worries and stresses of the day. Most importantly, exercise revitalises and energises the body as well as releases endorphins, the "feel good" hormones that induce relaxation, heighten pleasure, reduce the experience of pain and increase feelings of well-being.

Lower stress and boost immunity

One tremendous health benefit of lowering stress levels is a strong immune system. Almost every day, we hear about the importance of our immune system for our health, as a correctly functioning immune system provides protection against viruses, bacteria, and in some cases even cancer.

Effective defense against influenza is of great concern and interest to the general public. Every year up to one fifth of US residents will be infected by the seasonal influenza outbreak, and occasionally these may reach epidemic proportions.

Many people believe that the only way to defend themselves against a flu outbreak is to get a flu shot. In reality, it is very difficult to create an effective vaccine as the hallmark of influenza viruses is that they are constantly changing. However, in the following chapter, we will learn the seven effective steps for strengthening our immune system to keep infections away.

CHAPTER 5

The Pandemic Survival Kit: How to Supercharge Our Immune System

"You are what you eat, drink, breathe, think and do."
—Patrica Bragg

Viral Pandemics seem to be taking place with surprising regularity throughout world history. Reviewing human history, we see the deadly "H1" type flu virus striking several times in the last century. In 1918, 40 million people were killed in the Spanish flu outbreak. Thousands more succumbed to the Asian Flu of 1957 and the Hong Kong Flu of 1968.

Today with metropolitan cities across the world and global travels, there are more opportunities for viruses to spread at alarming speed. In view of the more recent SARS and swine flu outbreak, we see that even advanced medical technology is not effective in stopping the spread of virus.

However with prudence and precaution, we can protect our families and ourselves until the plague passes.

Whether it is the common flu or a global pandemic, the steps outlined in this chapter when carried out with vigilance are effective strategies for avoiding any viral infection.

> "During the last few years, the world has faced several threats with pandemic potential, making the occurrence of the next pandemic just a matter of time."
>
> The World Health Organization

First, we should establish that we catch the flu 'bug' not because we are sneezed at, or exposed to a contagious strain of flu virus. Germs are everywhere. Flu viruses can live for hours on supermarket trolleys, buttons in the elevators, door knobs, pens, computer keyboards, coffee mugs and other objects, so it is easy to come into contact with such viruses during daily life. Basically, germs can only infect us when our immune system is impaired. So boosting the immune function is therefore an essential step in safeguarding ourselves against the flu virus.

The rest of this chapter shows you how you can help your immune system to remain strong. We have already touched briefly on many of these steps in previous chapters, so you will find that much of this is familiar to you. Many of the tips for beating stress and for creating a healthy indoor environment will also aid you in strengthening your immune system. Here, we look at these building steps in greater detail.

7 Steps for boosting the immune function & beating the flu

Step 1) Minimize, manage, and eliminate stress.

Chronic stress, whether emotional or environmental, can suppress our immune function.

When we are stressed out, our immune system is impaired. Fostering good friendships, building emotionally fulfilling relationships, making little sacrifices to do something for the good of another, forgiving or simply saying we are sorry are all building blocks to a strong, resilient immune system. Meditative relaxation, prayers, taking deliberate breaks from work and doing more of the things we enjoy will help us manage daily stress and make us less susceptible to the flu.

Sleep deprivation is also a kind of stress to the body. A lack of high quality sleep will undermine our ability to resist a viral attack. Getting enough deep restorative sleep each day is preventive medicine.

Finally, take time to laugh. Laughter is indeed a remarkable medicine. A hearty laugh reduces stress, oxygenates the whole body and boosts the immune system. It also energizes the body, lifts the spirit and increases mental alertness and concentration.

Just like author Albert Hubbard said, "Don't take life too seriously. You'll never get out of it alive."

Step 2) Install an air ionizer

Installing a therapeutic, medical-grade air ionizer is an excellent defense against flu. A medical grade air ionizer generates small, biologically-active oxygen ions which help to deliver oxygen to the body at the cellular level.

Studies show that breathing small negative ions of oxygen, similar to those found in invigorating natural environments, stimulate the body's production of the antibody, immunoglobulin A, to fight infections.

This was conclusively proven in a six-year study undertaken by La Trobe University in Australia where research analyzed the effect of inhaling small negative air ions on the body's immune function.

Besides boosting the body's ability to fight off disease germs, oxygen ions have been shown to completely eliminate germs before we breathe them in.

The lethal effect of negative ions on a wide range of micro-organisms has long been noted by Professor A P Krueger during his decades of biological research. Negative ionization has since been used in various applications as an effective means of infection control. Continual research into air ionization as a potential solution to the spread of disease germs is currently being carried out.

The transmission of Salmonella enteritidis infection to humans through the handling and consumption of contaminated eggs has been a significant international public health issue.

A study undertaken by the USDA was performed on how effective negative ionization was at the eradication of Salmonella enteritidis from the air of hen houses.

The results of the study were dramatic in that the airborne bacterium of Salmonella was drastically reduced by ionization, resulting in reduced infections in egg-laying hens. The USDA released this statement:

"These results indicate that negative air ionization can have a significant impact on the airborne microbial load in a poultry house and at least a portion of this effect is through direct killing of the organisms."

In 1979, another interesting study was conducted by veterinary researchers in Helsinki, Finland, on the effectiveness of air ionization in the control of airborne transmission of the Newcastle Disease virus in chicken. Newcastle Disease is a serious and fatal contagious bird disease affecting many domestic and wild avian species. It is also transmissible to humans.

It was discovered that the airborne transmission of the Newcastle Disease virus was completely prevented with high negative ion density in the test room from a negative ion generator placed above the cage's wire-gauze roof. On the other hand, 90 percent of the chickens in the control group without air ionization contracted the virus transmitted through the air from diseased birds in a neighboring cage.

A year-long trial by the University of Leeds at St James Hospital in the UK, funded by a grant of £101,000 from NHS Estates, found that ionizers placed in the Intensive Care Unit significantly reduced infections by eliminating 100 percent of the highly resistant acinetobacter from the air. This pathogenic bacteria causes a wide variety of serious infections in humans, mostly in compromised patients and is resistant to most antibiotics.

Subsequent work by micro-biologists at Southampton University confirmed that negative ions have a lethal effect on exposed colonies of acinetobacter as well as e-coli, a common type of bacteria that can cause serious food poisoning in humans.

Hospitals are notorious places for picking up deadly infections caused by superbugs. In America, nearly two million hospital-acquired infections claim about 100,000 lives every year. Perhaps the answer to this problem is in creating an atmosphere of intensely electrified air that is extremely hostile to disease germs rather than the widespread use of stronger chemical antibacterial disinfectants which can lead to the emergence of yet another strain of superbugs.

Spending much of our lives in environments with ion-depleted air where infectious germs live longer means that diseases are able to spread more easily and rapidly. It is no surprise that we often pick up bugs in the office, school, childcare center, or any crowded place with dead stale air. Contagious influenza is quickly spread through the city as infectious germs are transported around in cars, buses, trains and planes.

Air ionizers are especially useful around young children, elderly people and those weakened from prolonged sickness or surgical procedures.

However, it is important that we choose a medically approved ionizer that has been certified to meet all safety standards. Many inferior ion generators produce ozone, which, being a lung irritant, can cause breathing difficulties and trigger allergic reactions including asthma.

A good negative air ionizer will help blood circulation, promote a positive mood, balance the body's blood chemistry to alleviate allergies and strengthen the immune system. It is invaluable weaponry against the flu bug and definitely a must-have in the event of a viral pandemic.

Step 3) Watch what you put into your body

It was recorded that the Biblical character, Daniel, had determined in his heart not to eat anything that would defile his body. If we have a high regard for our bodies, recognizing that it is the habitation of our souls, we would do well to be similarly resolved.

Processed food with dangerous chemical ingredients such as artificial flavors, colors, preservatives, chemical taste enhancers (such as MSG) and artificial sweeteners will suppress your immune function. Man-made chemicals and synthetic additives do not supply the required nutrients but increase the toxic load on our body, putting added strain on our excretory organs such as the liver and kidneys.

Deep fried foods and unnatural fats such as margarine and hydrogenated vegetable oils are high in trans fatty acids, which clog up our arteries and put undue stress on our body, undermining our immune system.

Sodas and energy drinks have an acidity level equal to that of car batteries and we certainly should not be putting such corrosive things into our bodies. Once we start eliminating harmful foods from our diets, we stop suppressing our immune system and allow the body's own healing potential to take over.

On the other hand, wholesome food including lots of fresh, clean fruits and vegetables are rich in nutrients and aid in strengthening our immune function.

Healthy oils are also essential. They include fish oil, cod liver oil, salmon oil, cold pressed coconut oil and olive oil. Garlic, onions, ginger, aloe, spirulina, berries, green tea and olive leaf extract are powerful anti-viral foods and should be included in our diet or through supplementation. Kimchi is a very palatable way of ingesting large amounts of raw garlic, ginger and onion, which are potent anti-viral foods.

Vitamin A, C, zinc and selenium also exhibit anti-viral properties and can be taken as supplements. However, take care to get the right dosage of any supplements by consulting your doctor or a naturopathic physician.

Step 4) Hydrate & oxygenate

Water is an important solvent that is necessary for carrying and delivering nutrients to, as well as removing waste from, all the cells in the body. Water is also essential for brain function. Soda, coffee and sugared drinks will not provide or replace the fluids necessary for body processes. It is important for us to keep our body hydrated by drinking sufficient water every day.

Difficulty in breathing and other respiratory ills, such as asthma and allergies, are often the result of the body's attempt to conserve water, as water is lost through exhalation. With reduced capability to breathe, we cannot oxygenate the body. Putting people on asthmatic drugs and inhalers and ignoring the need of the body for water, will in no way help the patient with his condition. With ample hydration, our respiratory system will be optimally supported.

Oxygen is essential for a strong functioning immune system. Bacteria, viruses, other harmful germs and even cancer cells are anaerobic and thrive in oxygen deprived environments.

As disease germs proliferate in an oxygen starved body, the immune system is undermined. By flooding our body with beneficial oxygen, we will become less susceptible to infections.

This is another reason why we should install air ionizers in our oxygen depleted homes and offices—to increase our oxygen intake effortlessly. Studies have shown that ionized oxygen molecules are readily absorbed into the body through inhalation, to provide a measurable boost to the body's immune system.

Step 5) Get some sunshine

The peak flu season occurs in the winter months due to the lack of sunshine and a deficiency in vitamin D. Sunlight exposure is necessary for the generation of vitamin D on the skin.

Studies have shown that people with the lowest vitamin D levels have significantly more recent colds or flu. The risk is even greater for those with chronic respiratory disorders like asthma.

Alarmingly, vitamin D deficiency is widespread in many industrialized countries where people have been taught to be afraid of the sun. Many people are so enshrined in the belief that sunlight is harmful that they lavishly cover themselves with sunscreen lotion. By doing that, they are depriving themselves of the healing properties of the sun.

There is much evidence showing that optimal levels of vitamin D are essential in reducing the risk of every disease, and especially cancers, diabetes, osteoporosis, colds, influenza, and other infectious diseases like tuberculosis. On the other hand, less than optimal vitamin D levels will significantly undermine the immune response, making us far more susceptible to contracting colds, influenza, and other respiratory infections.

Step 6) Get moving

A regular exercise program can significantly boost your immune system. Studies show that regular moderate exercise helps to prevent the common cold. A recent study also showed that subjects who exercised regularly demonstrated a 50 percentage increase in resistance to the flu.

Exercise improves the circulation of immune cells in the blood, also known as white blood cells. These cells are responsible for rounding up hostile pathogens throughout the body. With better blood circulation, the immune system becomes more efficient in dealing with a viral invasion.

Movement also helps to move the lymphatic fluid of the body. The job of the lymphatic fluid is to remove metabolic wastes as well as bacteria and viruses that have been captured by the body's defense system.

Unlike our circulatory system which has a heart to pump the blood throughout the body, the lymphatic fluid gets moved around only through physical movement. Thus, it is unwise to rest in bed all day long. Someone who is weakened by an infection, injury or chronic condition, should also attempt to move a little.

An easy and effective way to move the lymphatic fluid is simply deep abdominal breathing. Deep breathing of nature's fresh air also oxygenates the body to help fight infections.

Body Massage is a also great therapy for a sick person. Massaging increases blood and lymphatic fluid movement. In addition, the loving, physical touch involved in the massage induces the body to produce immune-boosting healing bio-chemicals to aid healing.

Hence, a regular exercise routine away from the stagnant, recycled indoor air, with the synergistic effect of gentle sunlight and fresh air will dramatically reduce the likelihood of acquiring an upper respiratory infection.

Caution however, should be taken not to physically overexert oneself while fighting an infection. Vigorous physical exercise during an illness can further stress the immune system and result in prolonging the sickness.

On the other hand, gentle movement such as stretching or walking keeps the lymph fluid moving to eliminate toxins and to ensure a healthy immune system.

Step 7) Observe personal hygiene

Hand washing is a personal hygiene habit that can help prevent the flu and other infections. Proper hand washing breaks the chain reaction of the spread of germs. Children especially, must be taught to avoid rubbing eyes and nose with dirty hands and to wash their hands before eating. We should also bathe daily and avoid physical contact with an infected person.

If there is flu pandemic, we should also by all means limit exposure to the virus. Flu virus is a respiratory virus. Once inhaled, it quickly overwhelms a weakened immune system and begins to multiply in the respiratory tract.

Some people try to keep out the virus with a face mask, but such masks are useless in protecting us against the virus because they are extremely small—the average virus is about one-hundredth the size of the average bacterium.

A good guideline would be to keep a distance of about five feet from anyone with the flu. In the case of a pandemic, we should avoid crowds and if possible stop travelling altogether.

A strong immune system protects us from all diseases

Our immune system is our first line of defense against everything from minor illnesses like a cold or the flu to life-threatening diseases like cancer. It is not possible to be optimally healthy if our immune system is compromised.

Destructive habits, chronic oxygen deprivation, dehydration, stressful lifestyles and toxin laden foods will make us easy victims to the next round of bugs that come along. Making changes towards a natural lifestyle by incorporating the steps outlined in this chapter will greatly enhance our resistance to infectious diseases.

Breathing air with an abundance of negative ions not only boosts the immune system, but also helps respiration, increases lung capacity and helps us enjoy invincible respiratory health. From the beginning of time, man has recognized the importance of fresh air for recovery from respiratory diseases.

In the next chapter, we will learn how to boost respiratory function to kick out asthma and allergies, the prevalent respiratory maladies of modern civilization.

CHAPTER 6

Defeating Asthma and Allergies

"Breathing is the first place, not the last, one should look when fatigue, disease or other evidence of disordered energy presents itself."
—Dr. Sheldon Hendler, The Oxygen Breakthrough

Here is an essay written by Jonathan, a sixth-grader.

"When I was four, I was diagnosed with asthma. It started with a runny nose. It remained runny for many days and I was picking up every cold that came around. If I started getting better, I would catch something else. A cough developed that lingered for a long while. The doctor prescribed some colorful cough liquids. I didn't get better. In fact I was rapidly going downhill. Later I developed chronic bronchitis, coughing day and night with high fevers.

A blood test showed that I was allergic to a lot of food including eggs, fish, nuts, milk and wheat. My mum religiously kept me from all these allergens but was not able to ward off my first attack. It came, the tightness in the chest, the wheeziness, the shortness of breath. The inhalers, the steroids and nebulizer became my constant companions.

I tried many therapies, but none of them worked. I was getting weaker day by day. I couldn't participate in the various pre-school events, the carnivals, the games and sports, and the parties. I liked school but I had to bring my own food and nebulizer to school. My condition worsened. I needed to be nebulized up to 4 times a day.

One day, I was wheezing so badly that the nebulizer gave no relief at all. I was quite out of breath. I was deadly pale and could not speak. When I finally reached the hospital, the doctors immediately doubled up the dosage of my medication. It was a miracle that I did not die from that life-threatening attack. I cried. I hated being sick all the time.

Later, I went to a natural doctor called a naturopath. She taught me how to clean myself, inside and outside. I had to do strange things like drinking lots of fresh juices, fast and breathe oxygen ions. For the rest of my life, I must eat healthy foods. Now, I am hale and hearty. I have superb stamina and great strength. I have learnt to unleash that POWER within me to heal myself. I have overcome asthma."

In childlike simplicity, Jonathan has kept journals about his sufferings and recovery in a few words. Those early distressing years have caused him to understand the value of feeling good and being able to breathe freely and that has led him to live a disciplined life, which includes making wise food choices every day.

While conventional medicine tells you that there is basically no cure for allergies and asthma and that you just have to manage it with medication, a lot of people have been able to throw out their inhalers and live allergy free lives by making changes to address the underlying causes of these conditions.

The link between allergies and asthma has been so totally substantiated that they are often discussed together. Up to 38 percent of patients with allergies also have asthma and 78 percent of those diagnosed with asthma have allergies.

There has been a global increase in the incidence of allergies and asthma. In America alone, 35 million people suffer from allergies amounting to 30 percent of the adult population and 40 percent of the child population. Allergies are more common than heart disease or diabetes, and 200 Americans now die from food allergies every year.

In 2010, more than 18.7 million people in the US were diagnosed with asthma and 7 million of those were children. Asthma is potentially life-threatening, with 3388 deaths from asthma in 2009 in the US despite more conventional treatments available.

There are different types of allergic reactions. There are reactions triggered by airborne particles that enter our airways. Those who are allergic to dust, pollen or chemical fumes react violently to exposure with coughing, sneezing, runny nose, wheezing, itchy, watery, and red eyes.

Allergic reaction to substances that come into contact with our skin may result in eczema and atopic dermatitis. An outbreak of hives on the skin is an allergic reaction to the food that has been ingested. Food allergy can also lead to constriction of the airways and eczema.

Allergies are signs of a toxic body with a malfunctioning immune system. A body that is clean and healthy internally will have the ability to neutralize offending invaders and react appropriately to these external reactive substances. Conversely, a toxic and compromised internal environment over-reacts to even the slightest exposure to foreign antigens with possible deadly results.

Let's look at the possible underlying causes of allergies and asthma and how we can eliminate or drastically reduce the symptoms.

Causes of allergies and asthma

1) A dysfunctional immune system

Allergy sufferers often have a compromised immune function with abnormal levels of a group of antibodies, known as immunoglobulin.

People with hypersensitive allergic reaction to allergens often exhibit elevated levels of immunoglobulin E (IGE) that triggers the release of large amounts of histamine upon exposure, resulting in immediate flare-ups. These people often suffer from conditions such as eczema, hay fever, allergic asthma and food allergies.

Similar reactions are also found in people who, rather than having too much immunoglobulin E (IGE) have too little immunoglobulin A (IGA)! Immunoglobulin A (IGA) protects the mucosal surfaces of the mouth, lung, throat and gastrointestinal linings from infections. People with a deficiency in IGA are often troubled by allergic disorders, recurrent infections, asthma, and food allergies.

Certain proteins disrupt the function of IGA and when ingested can cause damage to the gastrointestinal tract resulting in a condition known as leaky gut, whereby undigested proteins enter the blood stream through the gut lining evoking an intense defense response from the body. The body then goes into a hypersensitive state while it attempts to breakdown the undigested proteins resulting in symptoms of allergies.

Yeast, eggs, soy, gluten and milk are known culprits, especially gluten, which is a protein found in wheat and all associated grains, and casein which is the protein found in milk. Chronic stress also suppresses the secretion of IGA aggravating asthma and allergic conditions.

Many allergy sufferers have been tested and found to be intolerant of gluten and dairy products. By eliminating these and other gut damaging protein sources that cause disruption to the immune system, their allergic symptoms are markedly reduced. And as immune system is built up, it will be able to react appropriately to substances outside the body.

2) Air pollution

Over the last decade, a considerable number of scientific studies have reported adverse health effects associated with air pollution.

These effects include respiratory illness, impaired lung function and increased rate of mortality.

Clean natural air is composed mainly of nitrogen and oxygen, with small amounts of carbon dioxide and other gases such as argon, neon and helium. As we have seen in previous chapters, it is also highly electrified with a delicate balance of about five positive to four negative ions.

Pollution greatly distorts the composition of natural air with the addition of gaseous and particulate ingredients that pose health risks to everyone who breathes the air. Not only that, air in the city during rush hour has virtually no beneficial negatively charged air molecules, which have mainly been destroyed by pollutants from car exhaust.

An autopsy study done on more than a hundred young accident victims in Southern California found that almost all of them showed evidence of lung disease. Although few had outward signs of breathing disorders when alive, these young lifelong urban residents, aged between fourteen and twenty-five, had the lungs of much older people. There were early signs of chronic lung disease, including low-level bronchitis and chronic inflammation of the respiratory bronchioles.

This is important because it shows that chronic exposure to toxic fumes will catch up with us. Throughout human history, man has never before lived in the conditions that exist today. Although our bodies are extremely adaptive and have the capability to detoxify themselves, long-term exposure to polluted air will inevitably increase the burden on our systems and increase our risks to lung diseases.

A comprehensive study performed on populations living in different parts of the Los Angeles Basin showed that chronic exposure to a mixture of air pollutants results in less rapid growth of lung function in children and a greater rate of deterioration in adulthood.

Increased carbon dioxide content in the air results in more toxic pollen and increased incidences of hay fever.

In recent years, hay fever has increased in severity among susceptible individuals. Scientists attribute this to the elevated amount of pollen produced by plants in the cities. It is observed that a rise in atmospheric carbon dioxide levels from cars and coal-burning plants, as well as warming global temperatures have caused plants to produce more and nastier pollens.

An experiment carried out by researchers at the Harvard Medical School showed that the ragweed plant, which is one of the most allergy-provocative plant species, produces more than 61 percent more pollen when grown in an atmosphere of increased carbon dioxide levels!

Generally ragweed and other pollen producing weeds grow bigger and faster in and around urban areas and produce more pollen than in rural areas. This pollen is also more toxic in nature.

3) Ozone and its effects on asthmatics

There is a strong link between ozone levels in the ambient air and the severity of asthma. Asthma, the most common chronic respiratory disorder of childhood, is on the rise in industrialized nations. Ozone is an odorless, colorless gas comprising of three atoms of oxygen. While the ozone layer located in the upper atmosphere of the Earth protects us from harmful rays from the sun, ozone when located at ground level even in small amounts presents a serious air quality problem.

In the Earth's lower atmosphere, ozone is formed when chemical waste from cars, power plants and other sources react in the presence of sunlight.

Scientists studying the effects of ozone on the human body found that ozone irritates the respiratory system, reduces lung function, impairs the body's immune system and aggravates asthma. It can inflame and damage the lining of the lungs and cause long-term health problems.

Breathing smoggy air is particularly hazardous as smog contains an elevated level of ozone. Individuals who are susceptible to allergies and asthma should avoid staying outdoors for extended periods of time on smoggy summer days or during midday and afternoons when pollutant levels are generally highest.

Clearly, if the outside air is heavily polluted, opening the windows will not allow in the clean, fresh air that our bodies so urgently need for health. If you live in a heavily polluted urban area, you will need to consider an alternative method of providing yourself with clean air.

If shopping for an air cleaner, beware of ozone generators that are sold under the guise of 'air cleaners' and 'negative ionizers'. Marketing material promotes ozone generators and communicates the false and dangerous message that they are a safe option for controlling indoor air pollution.

Some vendors even state that their machines have been approved by government health departments for being a safe way to clean air in a confined space.

This is frightening. Nothing could be further from the truth. Health professionals have been rejecting this notion for almost 100 years. Ozone is a dangerous gas that should not be inhaled.

People with asthma and allergies can suffer greatly from these machines that promise to deliver 'cleaner air'. Ozone is emitted in large amounts that can trigger asthma attacks in sufferers. Opt for a therapeutic, medical-grade air ionizer instead that will not only keep the air clean and fresh but will also help to balance our internal chemistry to give us a sense of wellbeing.

4) Bad Indoor Air Quality

Modern people generally spend far more time indoors than past generations did. In addition, our modern indoor environments are more insulated and allergens such as molds and dust mites are propagated in our cooling and heating systems. Common household products are also major causes of indoor air pollution. Chemical aerosols, cleaning detergents and antibacterial cleaners are particularly linked with exacerbations of asthma in people afflicted with the disease.

Our homes may be free from disease-causing viruses and bacteria, but riddled with an assortment of dangerous chemical fumes that are known to depress the immune system and create sensitivity with repeated exposure.

This is particularly hazardous for young children whose height and play habits often cause them to be exposed to pollutants or aerosols that are heavier than air and tend to concentrate in their breathing zones.

Moreover, there is mounting evidence in support of the theory that early exposure to some dirt and germs actually programs the immune system to identify threats. It has been shown that small children with exposure to farm animals, pets and dust are protected from developing allergies later in life.

According to a 2002 study in *The New England Journal of Medicine*, kids who grow up in extremely clean homes are more likely to develop asthma and hay fever than kids who grow up on farms or in houses with some dirt. Children who are raised with pets, or who have older siblings, are also less likely to develop allergies, possibly because they are exposed to more bacteria.

Eliminating germs with harsh chemicals apparently does not provide long-term health benefits. We should let children be children and allow them to explore in natural environments and get dirty. Besides, old fashioned soap and water is sufficient to maintain sanitation in the home.

5) Overconsumption of sugar

Our nutrient-depleted urban diet is producing too many unhealthy, overweight individuals in cities throughout the world. According to the *Journal of The American Medical Association*, 68 percent of US adults are overweight or obese. Too much sugar, carbohydrates and unhealthy fats are consumed. People in the US eat about 150 pounds of sugar a year per person which translates to approximately 22 tablespoons of sugar every day.

In his medical practice, Dr Fred Pescatore MD, author of the Hampton's Diet, found that allergies and asthma are related to an overgrowth of the yeast fungus *Candida albicans* in the digestive tracts. He has found Candida to be a serious problem in most people with asthma and those who suffer from allergies.

In fact, his complementary medical approach to the treatment of allergies and asthma centers on the use of nutrition and supplementation to control the growth of this yeast in our bodies. His approach has helped many of his patients significantly reduce their medication, if not eliminate their symptoms completely within a relatively short time.

Candida is a fungus that is naturally present in our gastrointestinal tract. In normal circumstances, it is kept under control by the good bacteria in our gut. However, if we take too many courses of antibiotics, we eliminate the good bacteria that keep these fungi in check. Moreover, if we consume a diet that is high in sugar and simple carbohydrates, we create a highly acidic environment in which Candida thrives.

A study at the University of Sydney in Australia showed that dietary sugar is a contributing factor in the development of asthma. That is understandable considering that sugar feeds Candida as oxygen feeds fire. Overconsumption of sugar leads to the overgrowth of Candida which directly affects our gut health which in turn causes damage to the immune system.

It is said that a teaspoon of sugar can suppress the immune system by 56 percent and 2 teaspoons by 78 percent. Eliminating Candida is the cornerstone of Dr Pescadores's asthma and allergy cure and this is done through a very strict dietary protocol which includes the elimination of all forms of sugar.

Kicking out asthma and allergies for good

Allergies and asthma will greatly affect a person's quality of life. They can in fact be life threatening. Those at greatest risk are urban children. Asthma is the number one serious childhood disease in North America.

As we have seen, the underlying causes of asthma and allergies are damage to the external atmospheric environment and the internal environment of our gut. To ensure a permanent recovery and to prevent our children from developing these conditions, we need to restore our living environment to that in which we are naturally made to thrive. We also need to reverse the damage done to our gut and from there gradually build up our digestive function to improve nutrient absorption.

Having identified the culprits that have worked against our respiratory health, let us implement some practical steps, explained here in detail, which have been proven to kick out asthma and allergies so that we can say goodbye to breathlessness, wheezing and many other symptoms that have plagued us for so long.

Step 1) Breathe electrified air

We are one large alkaline battery. Don Tolman, also known as the "whole food medicine cowboy", wisely pointed out that if we hook ourselves to up an Electro-Cardiogram, we will output electricity just like a battery.

Healthy cells and tissues are made up of negatively-charged ionic particles, also called electrons. When an electron meets up with another electron, an electric current is conducted. This is known as electricity.

Negative ions in the air enhance that conductivity within our bodies. So it goes without saying that the more negatively charged our inputs are, the more energy we will have.

The air in our cities is depleted of negative electrical charges. The naturally occurring negative ions in our air are rapidly consumed by the overwhelming amount of pollutants from our roads and highways. The urban concrete jungle with its lack of natural vegetation also inhibits the natural generation of negative ions.

As we have seen in previous chapters, negative ions are natural air cleaners. They transfer their electric charge to contaminants, clumping them together and causing them to fall out of the atmosphere. Without these air cleaning ions, particulates and fumes in our cities drift around indefinitely in the air currents afflicting all who breathe them in.

The problem with city air is the dominance of positive ions in its composition. And positive ions are known to make asthma victims worse. Positive ion winds, also stigmatized as "Witches Winds", such as the Chinook Wind in Calgary and the Santa Ana Winds in South California are known to coincide with increased incidences of asthma attacks.

Since it is not practical for most of us to leave the cities and move to the mountains, we have to take precautions to minimize exposure to polluted air and incorporate lifestyle changes to help us cope with modernity. We can and have to live healthily in an increasingly unnatural world.

We read in Chapter Three of the many things we can do to improve our indoor environment and increase the electrical charge of the air in our homes or offices. We can grow indoor plants or install a pretty water fountain. However for anyone who is dealing with chronic allergies and asthma, a therapeutic medical-grade air ionizer that generates massive amounts of negative ions continuously, could better provide the therapeutic effect necessary for healing.

Negative ions improve respiratory function

When it comes to the optimal functioning of our lungs, little hairs known as cilia keep the bronchial tubes and air passageways clear by moving in a sweeping motion. These form the first level of filtration which cleans the air we inhale of dust and pollen and other matter that should not reach the lungs. They work with mucus and remove tiny particles from the airways and lungs.

Negative ions have been found to speed up the rate of the movement of the cilia, which normally sweep at 900 beats per minute. Exposure to positive ions has been found to slow them to around 600 beats per minute.

When Dr Albert P Krueger and Dr Richard F Smith exposed tracheal tissue to negative ions they discovered that the cilia beat was increased to 1200 a minute.

Subjected to tobacco smoke, which absorbs negative ions, the cilia slow down. This indicates that smoking and all forms of pollutants that absorb air ions will adversely affect the ability of the cilia to block offending substances from entering our lungs, resulting in irritation of the airways which react with coughing and mucus production.

Interestingly, however, the scientists found that an overdose of negative ions neutralizes the effect of smoke on the cilia. It goes to show that air electricity can protect us from the effects of airborne particles by enabling the cilia to work more efficiently.

In his treatment of burn patients with negative ion therapy, Dr Kornblueh observed that those patients with chronic bronchitis or asthma reported that the therapy helped them to breathe better. This accidental discovery led him to start investigating the effects of ions on respiratory problems.

Dr Kornblueh's research at the University of Pennsylvania's Graduate Hospital found that exposure to negative ions helped patients who suffer from hay fever and or asthma. In fact, 63 out of every 100 experienced partial to total relief.

Many respected medical institutes have performed research on how negative ions can mitigate the effects of asthma and allergies. Thirty years of analysis at the Pavlov Institute in Russia discovered that 85 percent of asthmatics gained relief from being exposed to negative air ions. In addition hay-fever sufferers, people with skin rashes and sinusitis also benefited.

St Bartholomew's Hospital in London and The University of Canberra in Australia have also undertaken extensive research that has shown that improvement in lung capacity and relief from asthma symptoms can be achieved quite rapidly with exposure to small negative air ions.

In an Australia-wide survey of users of a leading medically approved air ionizer carried out in 2009, 93 percent of the respondents who bought the ionizer specifically to assist them gain relief from asthma reported an improvement in their condition, which they attributed to the use of the ionizer.

Of those who had purchased the ionizer to assist with hay fever and allergies, 89 percent had gained benefit and improvement in their condition as a result of their use of the ionizer. A few claimed that the generator had cured them completely.

At a Jerusalem hospital, doctors performed a series of tests on thirty-eight infants who suffered from respiratory problems. These babies were between two and twelve months old. They were divided into two equal groups and housed in two different wards. In one ward, an air ionizer was left operating while the other was kept as a control group in a ward without an ionizer.

The researchers reported that the infants treated with negative ions seemed to recover faster from asthma and bronchitis without the need for drugs. They were less prone to relapses and also did not cry as often and as loudly. As the subjects were all babies, the doctors dismissed the possibility of a placebo effect.

Breathing negative ions also stimulates the body to increase production of immunoglobulin A (IGA) which regulates allergy responses and guards against respiratory infections

Negative ion therapies are effective in providing relief from asthma and allergies due to the ions' ability to help the body modulate immune response, and to break down stress hormones that aggravate symptoms.

Those of us who have been chronically plagued with congestion and have forgotten what it is like to be able to breathe freely would appreciate the good feeling associated with the relief that comes from breathing negative ions. The doctors involved in Dr Kornblueh's project commented that the subjects would come in sneezing, eye watering, nose itching and worn out from lack of sleep, but just fifteen minutes in front of the ion generator and they would feel so much better that they did not want to leave.

Step 2) Ensure optimal hydration

In other words, drink enough water. Dr F Batmanghelidj MD, author of *Your Body's Many Cries for Water* asserts that allergies and asthma are directly linked to water deficiency in the body. The allergies are our bodies' built-in drought management program.

Water is essential to life. It regulates body temperature, carries nutrients to every cell, removes toxins, maintains the body's delicate PH balance, cushions joints and is needed for a host of other physiological functions.

We become dehydrated when the body does not get enough water to carry out its work. Water is lost through breathing as exhaled water vapor. In order to conserve water, the body releases histamine to incite spasm in the bronchial tubes, resulting in symptoms of asthma and allergies. As a clinician, Dr Balmanghelidj has helped many patients to eradicate asthma with water alone.

As asthma and allergies are complications of not drinking water regularly, his advice is to drink enough water daily to achieve colorless urine. Avoid alcoholic or caffeine-containing beverages and sodas, which do not quench the body's need for water but actually cause the kidneys to draw on the body's water reserve to flush out the unwanted substances contained in these less-than-healthful drinks.

Former President Ronald Reagan's personal doctor, Ralph Bookman M.D. has long been promoting hydration as a means of relieving asthma and allergy symptoms. He explained that adequate fluids are necessary to expel bronchial mucous secretions. In an interview, Dr Bookman said, "Liquids make mucus liquid. Liquids are medications." He recommends ten glasses of liquid each day for his patients.

Step 3) Boost the body's immune system with nutrition and dietary changes

To eradicate asthma and allergies, we have to remove the underlying causes of a compromised gastrointestinal system which disrupts the immune function and do everything we can to fortify our immune system.

Besides breathing fresh air that is electrically charged, we can achieve this through dietary changes. Here are some tangible and practical tips that we can implement straightaway to boost our immune system and to kick out asthma and allergies for good:

a) Avoid sugar

Eliminating sugar from our diet is key to restoring the body balance of bacterial flora, which has a direct correlation on asthma, allergies and food sensitivity. This can be extremely difficult as sugar is in almost everything we consume. Besides candy, cake, ice-cream, cookies, puddings and soda, it is also contained in almost all prepackaged foods, canned foods, boxed foods and condiments.

As you read the food labels, look out for these disguises of sugar: high-fructose corn syrup, fructose, sucrose, cane sugar, rice syrup, sorbitol, invert sugar, brown sugar, xylitol, mannitol, concentrated fruit juice and hydrogenated starch. White flour products such as white bread, pastries and pasta are simple carbohydrates which convert into sugar soon after ingestion and should also be avoided. Eliminating sugar can be extremely challenging for many people as sugar has an addictive effect. One way to overcome sugar addiction is to substitute sugar dense foods with nutrition dense foods. Most sugar craving is the result of deficiencies in essential nutrients. So, as the body starts to receive the needed nourishments, cravings for sweet empty foods will cease. Another way to control sugar addiction is through visualization.

Imagine your favorite pizza crawling with obnoxious worms and maggots and immediately it will seem very much less appealing.

b) Eliminate wheat and dairy products

Gluten in wheat and other grains such as barley, oats, rye and buckwheat, as well as casein in milk products, are proteins that can disrupt the function of IGA in the intestinal tract, resulting in a leaky gut. By eliminating these gut damaging proteins, we can help stop the assaults and allow the immune system to heal.

Wheat is one of the most widely eaten cereals and is found in an enormous number of foods. Breads, cookies, cakes, crackers, noodles, pastries, pancake, pasta, pies, pretzels and waffles are obvious wheat products. However, wheat is also hiding in fillers in sausages, hamburgers, meat loaf, potato croquettes and fish cakes. The effect of gluten on gut health is widely-known, and we can see that through the emergence of a host of gluten free products.

Eliminating dairy products may be that one factor which will help you get rid of your symptoms permanently. Many people are intolerant of milk without even knowing it. It is advisable to avoid all forms of milk, whether dried, evaporated or skimmed, as well as cheese. Milk is also used in the making of ice-cream, sherbet, creamed soups, puddings, protein powdered drink mixes and energy bars.

c) Consume lots of good fats

People with asthma and allergies must increase their intake of good fats from food sources rich in essential fatty acids such as fish, chia seeds, nuts, olive oil, coconut oil and macadamia nut oil. This is because good fats are anti-inflammatory.

Bad fats on the other hand promote inflammation and are in almost every processed food as trans fats or partially hydrogenated oils. Vegetable oil such as soy or corn oil that is usually used for cooking is extremely unhealthy. This is because they are very unstable and turn rancid quickly at high temperatures. Coconut oil and macadamia nut oils are the recommended oils for cooking as they have high smoking points and do not oxidize easily.

d) Get your nutrients from natural whole foods

The cornerstone of good health is proper nutrition. With a high functioning digestive system, we will be able to get the nutrients we need to normalize and fortify our immune system to deal with asthma and allergies. Choose locally grown organic whole foods rather than chemically treated commercial produce.

Pesticides are estrogenic and neurogenic and when ingested will create great internal disharmony, impairing the immune system.

Be sure to include beta carotene rich foods in your diet every day as these are known to promote lung function. These include carrots, kale, mustard green, sweet potatoes, goji berries and spirulina.

Vitamin C dense foods are also important for people who are prone to allergies and hay fever. Citrus fruits, kiwi fruits and all kinds of berries are great sources of vitamin C.

Asthmatics and allergy sufferers are also frequently deficient in important minerals such as zinc and magnesium and these are to be obtained from a diet comprising of a wide variety of fresh whole foods.

In contrast to synthetic vitamins and minerals, nutrients from unprocessed real foods are readily assimilated into our bodies for they are delivered as a nutrient complex with all the co-enzymes and co-factors necessary for absorption.

Step 4) Try an enema

In seeking an effective treatment for their son's asthma, Jonathan's parents had flipped and floundered around, in and out of all forms of therapies that were claimed by their promoters as "the cure". They realized that the idea of "a pill for every ill" is much flawed and true healing can only begin when we understand how our body works and respect the laws of nature.

Besides putting into practice the steps outlined in this chapter, incorporating improvements in the air, water and food that are taken into the body daily, Jonathan was tremendously helped by what seemed a rather peculiar therapy, the coffee enema.

The coffee enema is actually an important aspect of the famous Gerson Therapy that has helped thousands to reverse even serious degenerative and life-threatening conditions. Its effectiveness stems from the fact that the proper removal of toxins and debris from the colon is absolutely essential in all conditions of disease and ill health.

Jonathan found that the enema relieved his asthma attacks and gave him a sense of wellbeing. In fact, the effect was almost immediate. He had found that he always could breathe much better after the procedure. Even though the boy has been asthma free for a long time now, he still asks for his regular enemas, not so much for crisis management, but for that periodic gentle detoxification and the maintenance of good health.

For every ailment we have, the whole body must be treated, because every individual organ is an integral part of the whole person.

There is never any manifestation of pain or ailment in any single part of the body, in which the entire system is not involved.

In the next chapter, we shall turn our attention to one of the most shocking health issues facing the modern world—the risk from our polluted environment to our children, not only of asthma and allergies as described in this chapter, but of neurological disorders.

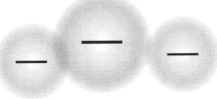

CHAPTER 7

How to Save Our Children from the 4-A Disorders

"Where there is great love there are always miracles."
—Willa Cather

The 4-A disorders, autism, ADHD (attention deficit hyperactivity disorder), asthma and allergies are now recognized by medical scientists, particularly in the industrialized nations, as reaching epidemic proportions among children.

What can we do to stem the tide?

What happened to our children?

The following short extract was written by a young student teacher who was just starting out on her teaching career in a boys' school in Singapore. Under the government's "many helping hands" approach, a number of children with special needs are integrated into the mainstream schools to provide opportunities for meaningful interactions and acceptance of these children in society. Many students are admitted as normal children but subsequently diagnosed as having learning or behavioral disorders.

"Throughout the music lesson, Joseph was in a world of his own. I was told he was autistic and I was asked to be watchful. He was quietly doodling, oblivious to all that was going on around him. I tried to engage him by speaking gently with him. There was no response, no eye contact.

We carried on with the class activities. Songs, movement and stories— what fun. Suddenly, an eerie unearthly sound escaped Joseph's lips. The singing stopped abruptly and all eyes were turned in his direction. Joseph had started to strip himself naked.

I rushed over to clothe him. "You mustn't do that, you are in school." I told him softly. He calmed down and allowed me to button up his shirt. I had barely turned to go when I saw a table flung across the room. He screamed and turned hysterical. At this point, another teacher came in and helped. I stood there, shaken and very broken hearted.

At that particular all-boys' school where I was contracted to teach, up to 10 percent of the students had been diagnosed with some kind of learning and behavioral disorder including Autism and ADD or ADHD (attention deficit disorder, and attention deficit hyperactivity disorder).

Special programs with specialized teachers were implemented to help these children "catch up", but progress was painfully slow. The following year, 12 percent of the new intake was classified as "special needs" kids. The school counselors and allied teachers were stressed out and overworked.

A colleague of mine, who had been transferred from another school, told us that up to 15 percent of the student body of his previous school had "special needs". Asthma and allergies were also prevalent in our student population. Pale kids with scaly skin and diverse sensitivities dot the general assembly.

This is a worrisome trend and what I had experienced and seen as a very junior teacher was based on just my limited exposure to the educational sector in tiny Singapore. In fact, I was to find out later that childhood learning and behavioral disorders together with asthma and allergies have literally exploded into a full blown epidemic."

The world is seeing a disturbing emergence of childhood conditions of unprecedented proportions. Developmental learning & behavioral disorders in the form of Autism, Asperger's Syndrome, Attention Deficit Disorder (ADD/ADHD) and Hyperactivity have invaded many households, claiming the bodies and minds of our children.

The number of children receiving special education services continues to rise steeply. Dr Andrew Wakefield, stated in his book *Callous Disregard* that if autism does not affect your family now, it is almost a mathematical certainty that it will in the future.

The current rate of such disorders is undeniably alarming. Over the past 20 years, we have seen a 1500 percent to 6000 percent increase in autism in the US, supposedly the world's most advanced nation, with an estimate of 1.5 million American children being diagnosed with autism-spectrum disorders.

ADHD has increased by 400 percent; now 3.5 million US children have ADHD. We also see an exponential increase in the number of incidences of childhood allergies and asthma. Childhood asthma has increased 300 percent, with 6 million children being diagnosed with asthma. Asthma deaths have increased by 56 percent despite the better care for acute asthmatic crisis. Allergies in children have grown by 400 percent with an estimated 200 deaths from allergies every year.

Generally, children with learning and behavioral disorders are usually also plagued with various forms of allergies. Experts point out the connections between autism, ADHD, asthma and allergies and term them collectively as the childhood epidemics of the 4-A disorders.

They have the same root causes which are environmental assaults on the yet immature immune and gastrointestinal systems of the young.

Causes of childhood 4-A epidemics

Environmental pollution

Dr Kenneth Bock in his book *Healing the New Childhood Epidemics*, explains that catastrophic changes in the environment of our children accounts for the skyrocketing incidences of childhood disorders. Widespread pollution and the prevalence of toxins in our air, food and water have contributed significantly to this trend.

It is estimated that close to 300,000 tons of heavy metals annually are released into the atmosphere due to worldwide coal and fuel oil combustion as well as industrial processes involved in the mining and refining of metal-containing ores. Other industries also release large amounts of brain damaging substances into the air.

The US Environmental Protection Agency identifies one third of these industrial byproducts as hazardous air pollutants. They include arsenic, beryllium, cadmium, cobalt, chromium, mercury, manganese, nickel, lead, antimony, selenium, uranium and thorium.

Of these, mercury from coal-burning plants, lead from metal processing facilities and battery manufacturers, and diesel exhaust fumes are particularly damaging to the nervous systems of fetuses and young children, resulting in lowered IQs and learning problems.

Open smokestacks in Leominster, Massachusetts for instance, have brought into existence shockingly high number of "autism clusters".

These pollutants, dispersed into the air as invisible particles, are blown by the winds and widely circulated. They also rain down from the atmosphere in sufficient quantities into water bodies to enter into aquatic plants and the food chain.

Nutritional deficiencies

A lack of essential nutrients in the daily diet of our children is also a factor in the exponential increase in the prevailing childhood conditions among our young population. The standard American diet has infiltrated even eastern cultures and has spread to the cities of the world.

High consumption of white flour, soda and processed food, which are devoid of essential nutrients, thwarts the development of young bodies and minds.

As a result our children suffer chronic nutritional deficiencies, and their bodies are not able to properly protect, detoxify and repair themselves.

Childhood vaccinations

Another factor, though still controversial, has been brought to the attention of the public since renowned public health advocates began to write extensively about it. The increased number of childhood vaccinations has been implicated in the tidal wave of childhood disorders in recent years.

A form of mercury preservative called thimerosal is used in the manufacture of vaccines to prevent bacterial contamination. Mercury is a very effective antibacterial but is especially damaging to the brain and human nervous system.

Only in 2001 was thimerosal gradually phased out of vaccine because of the outcry of thousands of concerned parents. However, much damage has already been done. Even so, flu shots still contain mercury and are recommended to children above six months old, as well as pregnant mothers.

Additionally, immune adjuvants, which are agents added to invoke an intense immune response, contain aluminum compounds which are also very harmful to the brain. Moreover, the number of immunizations has increased to twenty or more within the first eighteen months of a baby's life. In excess and given within a short period of time, the viral materials also add to the toxic load of the child.

The cumulative toxicity of the vaccines administered within a short period of time is a tremendous assault to the child's immature immune system, leading to the onset of childhood asthma, allergies or behavioral and learning disorders.

How to protect our children from these childhood epidemics

Step 1) Reduce their exposure to environmental toxins

A large part of the problem lies in the widespread exposure to environmental toxins in our air, water and food. Our homes should be sanctuaries of love where our children can be free to explore and grow in total safety. They should be given the environmental and nutritional support necessary for their overall development.

Enriching the indoor air with an abundance of healthful negative ions takes care of the hazards associated with positive ion poisoning and airborne allergens. Install a therapeutic negative ionizer and run it throughout the day.

As we have seen, negative ions also destroy harmful pathogens and boost the child's immunity against infections. Inhaled negative ions readily enter the bloodstream to invoke a natural immune response with increased secretion of IgA.

Wounds and cuts are also less likely to get infected in a bacteria-free atmosphere. Injuries, cuts and scratches sustained through falls and knocks heal rapidly and often with little scarring.

We have seen how positive ions make breathing more difficult and reduce the body's ability to absorb oxygen; and how negative ions help breathing and improve oxygen absorption. As such the negative ionizer is important weaponry against asthma and allergies.

Liquid and aerosol detergents that we use liberally every day to protect our families from germs are great causes of indoor pollution.

These chemicals are marketed as anti-bacterial and effective in eliminating microbes. However, the chemical molecules emitted by these household cleaners are so minute and light that they remain airborne.

Children and toddlers are closer to the floor and often explore on all fours, thus routinely ingesting and inhaling toxic chemicals used in cleaning products, and for long periods of time. Their bodies will, sooner or later, react to the chemicals.

It is noteworthy that chemicals that produce allergies are different from natural irritants such as pollen. For natural substances, the healthy body is able to use its array of antibodies to attack the offending protein and neutralize its chemically active "surface".

In other words, it has protein-specific antibodies that defend itself against foreign antigens at the location of entry such as the eyes, nose and lungs.

However, the body cannot protect itself against harmful gases and chemicals as they do not possess proteins in their composition. A healthy body can naturally deal with dust mites and pollen, but is vulnerable to chemicals.

So, one of its defense mechanisms is to shut down the lungs to prevent noxious gases and chemical from entering the system and injuring its delicate cells, in particular the brain cells, resulting in symptoms of allergies, respiratory difficulties or a full blown asthma attack.

Asthma and allergies are conditions of a weakened body with a compromised immune system, the result of repeated assault from exposure to chemicals.

As the body becomes increasingly incapable of dealing with foreign particles, autoimmune disorders ensue. As such we should always go for "all natural products" that contain no chemicals.

Step 2) Encourage them to drink sufficient water

Chronic dehydration is also a cause of asthma and allergies, especially in children. Dr E. Batmanghelidi, author of *Your Body's Many Cries for Water*, explains that asthma and allergies are important indicators of dehydration in the body.

Breathing itself results in a loss of water. The winter steam that we see when we breathe out in cold weather is water that is leaving our lungs as we breathe. Since we breathe about 720 times an hour, we can imagine the amount of water loss through breathing alone.

Children need water for cell growth and 75 percent of the cell volume during growth is water. When we fail to replace water loss, the body's water conservation mechanism is activated. Bronchial tubes constrict to minimize water loss during breathing. As children's bronchial trees are smaller and less rigid they exhibit shortness of breath and develop asthma more readily.

Soda and other manufactured beverages cannot replace the water needs of the human body. Simple, plain water is what our body is designed to receive. As a guide, Dr Batmanghelidi recommends that a person takes in half of his body weight in ounces of water each day. A 60 pound child will need about 30 ounce of water a day to maintain optimal hydration.

Step 3) Incorporate healing, nutrient-rich foods into their diet

We have to be even more vigilant now than ever before because of the sneaky way synthetic food additives are ending up in our children's food, even commercial baby foods. The nutritional value of school lunches is also questionable.

A rule of thumb is to provide fresh organic fruits and vegetables for our families. Entice children with brightly colored, delicious seasonal fruits and vegetables that are abundant in nutrients, anti-oxidants and immune-enhancing vitamins. Avoid commercially-raised meats as they are full of synthetic hormones and antibiotics.

A glass of yummy green smoothie first thing in the morning delivers a generous supply of chlorophyll, vitamins, minerals, enzymes and antioxidants into our children's bodies providing the necessary building blocks for growth and development.

Victoria Boutenko, bestselling author and raw food expert tells how her whole family's health was turned around by healing raw foods when conventional medicines failed.

Her daughter was born with asthma and allergies and would often cough heavily through the night while her son had diabetes. She made popular the green smoothie as an easy and pleasant way of consuming more living plant life.

A child with an established diagnosis of ADD/ADHD or other learning disabilities, even if his condition is improved by the use of conventional medication, can gain added benefits from the following tips: stick to a nutritional plan which includes a natural whole foods and sugar-free diet; identify and eliminate food allergies; avoid processed foods and especially foods with additives, colors and preservatives.

Step 4) Administer vaccination within reasonable safety boundaries

Dr Kenneth Bock recommends safer vaccination, administered properly without thimerosal to healthy children over an extended time period. No vaccination is completely free of risk. If an elder sibling has a 4-A disorder, extra caution should be exercised when immunizing your child. In addition:

- Postpone the vaccination if your child is ill, or was ill within the past week
- Do not vaccinate your child if he is experiencing an allergic response until all allergic symptoms have cleared
- Insist on vaccinations without thimerosal
- Monitor your child for adverse reactions after the immunization. Contact your doctor immediately if there are any symptoms of illness

- Breast feed your infant to confer immunity while his/her immune system is still underdeveloped

Step 5) Ensure a continuous supply of electrified air

European studies concluded that excess serotonin inhibits the flow of information in the brain, interfering with the ability to learn. Conversely, negative ions, which nullify the effects of excess serotonin, aid learning.

A top boys' school in Singapore instituted the practice of releasing the students for 15 minutes in the middle of the school day, for the sole purpose of romping in the open air outside. The boys are reported to return better composed and ready to learn.

A study in 1982 found that when a drug was administered that reduced serotonin levels, IQ and behavior both improved in autistic children. The hormone serotonin also plays a major role in moods and behavior.

When there is excess serotonin being produced (and not broken down by negative ions) this imbalance can result in depression, obsessive compulsive disorder, obesity and aggression.

Bullying in school has been attributed to the amount of time students spend indoors, crammed together in assembly areas, libraries, locker rooms, computer rooms, school buses and indoor sport halls, breathing in excessive positive ions for hours.

As early as 1975, Altman's Environment and Social Behavior study discovered that altering the electrical conditions of the room could have a positive effect on the performance of school children. Error rates were reduced and mental functioning increased with the addition of negative ions to the environment. A group of kindergarten teachers reported a considerable increase in concentration, calmness and reduced absenteeism when an ionizer was used in their classrooms.

According to Pierce J Howard, author of *The Owner's Manual for the Brain: Everyday Applications from Mind-Brain Research* and director of Research for Applied Cognitive Sciences in Charlotte, negative ions can help us to think better. "Generally speaking, negative ions increase the flow of oxygen to the brain; resulting in higher alertness, decreased drowsiness and more mental energy."

In 1984, a study on the effectiveness of negative ions on mental performance was conducted. It was found that exposure to negative air ions supported better communication between the brain hemispheres in learning-disabled children.

The study showed conclusively that negative ions improve the cognitive abilities of mentally handicapped children, as well as the abilities of normal children. The published results indicated that negative ions enhanced performance in the order of 8.4 percent for normal children, 23.6 percent for the learning-disabled and 54.8 percent for the mildly retarded.

ADD/ADHD and learning disabilities are usually found together. Poor communication between the right and left brain hemispheres are at the core of these disorders. High levels of serotonin are almost always present in children with learning disabilities or ADHD.

As we have already discussed in several places in earlier chapters, poor air quality with an excess of positive ions is the most frequent cause of abnormally high levels of serotonin. Revitalizing the indoor space with negative air electricity creates an environment that is conducive to learning.

Breathing beneficial negative ions persistently, over time on a regular basis, helps correct the internal chemistry of the child and consequently creates positive learning experiences for him.

A Negative Air Ionizer—A student's best friend

Sharon was a special needs teacher and had a cold. She didn't want to infect the children with germs, so took a negative ionizer to school with her. It turned out to be one of the best special needs teaching days she had ever had.

Her pupils were lovely children, who happened to all have learning and behavioral problems. This made teaching them a particularly fulfilling job but it was also very challenging.

Sharon knew that the ionizer was capable of cleaning the air of bacteria, so decided that she'd save the children from having to endure the inconvenience and discomfort of getting the cold. The ionizer delivered further results by enabling the children who found it difficult to concentrate to focus and cooperate with her requests.

The ionizer was so effective that she purchased one for the classroom.

Apparently, negative air ions at therapeutic doses moderate hyperactivity, produce a calming effect, and promote concentration and learning in children with learning and behavioral disorders.

Love makes all the difference

"Special needs" children can be very creative and imaginative thinkers with good intentions, but have trouble getting along with their peers and teachers. Later in life, that can translate into difficulties in work management, relationships, drug and alcohol dependence, depression, despair and crime.

By addressing metabolic and environment issues, we tackle the root of these prevailing childhood problems and are assured of a good chance of success in comparison to the use and reliance on prescriptive drugs and stimulants with all the undesirable side effects which may include hostility, aggressive behavior, fatigue, depression, sexual dysfunction and suppression of creativity.

A supportive group of parents, teachers and friends who value these children as individuals, and a disciplined lifestyle which includes nutritionally-dense whole foods and a constant supply of fresh negative ion-rich air can definitely help them along the way in their learning journey and through their growing up years.

Learning and behavioral disabilities and other childhood diseases are far from being primarily genetic. Allergies affect one third of our children, asthma one fourth. ADHD afflicts one in ten and autism one in hundred.

Such epidemics are the result of the assaults of recent environmental changes on genetic vulnerabilities. The greatest protection we can offer a child is an environment charged with the essence of fresh air and with the most generous and powerful form of love, the love of a parent for a child and all that entails.

The legacy that we can leave our children is wisdom to live a good life. This cannot be found in books alone, for in fact we have too many books in this world and not all contain sound knowledge. Wisdom is passed to the next generation as we walk our walk each day, caring for ourselves and nature and appreciating the things that are truly important and necessary in life, one of which is fresh electrified air.

The movie Food Matters recently presented us with the staggering and shocking statistics on preventable deaths due to hospital stays and medical care. It was reported that annually in America up to 225,000 deaths are associated with surgery procedures and other errors, hospital infections and adverse drug reactions. It appears that hospital can be a very dangerous place!

However, in the event of a hospital stay being necessary, the healing powers of air electricity can be harnessed and practical precautionary steps can be taken to minimize treatment complications and shorten recovery time. We shall examine this and look into how we can survive a hospital stay in the next chapter.

CHAPTER 8

How to Minimize Surgery Complications and Shorten Recovery Time

"90 percent of our metabolic oxygen comes from breathing.
10 percent comes from food."
—Dr Gabriel Cousins

Dr Rehn and the red smoke of Ettenheim

In the early 1950s, a peculiar phenomenon was described by a brilliant surgeon and teacher, Dr E. Rehn, in his account of the Red Smoke of Ettenheim and how it might have saved his patients. Dr Rehn was an accomplished neurosurgeon who worked in the neighboring towns of Freiburg and Ettenheim near Munich in Southern Germany.

Munich was often plagued by the notorious seasonal wind known as the Foehn, which would bring a massive amount of positive air ions. Post-surgery deaths due to blood problems in and around Munich were alarmingly common. Profuse bleeding requiring heavy transfusion and thrombosis were frequent and often resulted in death. Thrombosis is a condition when the patient's weak body mysteriously develops blood clots that travel through arteries to clog a vital organ.

However, when Dr Rehn was appointed as Head of Neurosurgery at Ettenheim, just 25 miles from Freiburg, he noticed that patients who were in the Ettenheim hospital were recovering better than the ones in the Freiburg hospital. He could not imagine what the difference could be. Maybe it was the food or the water that made such a difference, but whatever it was, the patients in Ettenheim fared well on it.

Something that the nurses in Ettenheim hospital had to contend with was the red smoke that was emitted by a local factory. In fact, there was so much of it that it stained the clothing of the town's inhabitants—which infuriated them. A thick red smoke lay over the town particularly when there was no wind. The local population petitioned for something to be done about the smoke and the factory added smoke filters to their chimneys.

Dr Rehn then noticed that the death rate in Ettenheim rose until it was much the same as that in Freiburg.

At the time when the red smoke had been present, an air analysis had been carried out by a Dr W Spitzer, who noted that there was a large negative electrical charge in the air. Apparently, the red smoke came from furnaces that burned materials high in radioactivity, resulting in the by-production of a large volume of negative air ions.

Dr Rehn's conclusion was that the red smoke, so heartily disliked by the inhabitants of Ettenheim, had in fact had life-giving properties, which could only be explained by its high level of negative ions.

The winds, the moon and surgery

Doctors who live in the areas where the Foehn winds pass with their strong charge of positive ions avoid surgery during the time of the wind. It has become clear to them that a patient is more likely to die when the wind blows, either on the operating table or just after it.

When the moon is full, or nearly full, the interaction of the negatively charged moon with the ionosphere about seventy-five miles above the Earth causes the number of positive ions close to the Earth's surface to increase. The ionosphere is a layer of electrically charged air and particles that envelop the Earth and protect it from much of the Sun's harmful radiation.

Countless scientific studies conducted across the world demonstrate that the lunar cycle affects human behavior. The word "lunatic" was coined from vast accumulated folk wisdom based on the frequently observed connection between bizarre human behavior and the time of the full moon.

Excessive atmospheric positive ions during the time of the full moon cause the overproduction of the stress neuro-hormone serotonin resulting in mental and physical dis-equilibrium. The already mentally disturbed may exhibit restlessness and some may even become irrationally violent.

Excessive positive ions also have a stimulating effect with deadly repercussion for bleeding patients. Dr Shealy, head of the Pain Clinic and a neurosurgeon at La Crosse, Wisconsin, ran a survey among fellow doctors about the amount of severe bleeding that occurred in patients when surgery was undertaken during the time of the full moon. It was also noted that there were more requests for blood transfusions around the time of the full moon or during the two days after it.

Dr Edson Andrews in Tallahassee, Florida noted that 82 percent of patients who had excessive bleeding problems had undergone surgery during the time of the full moon. He ordered that no surgery should take place during that time.

Medical application of negative ionization

Negative ions reduce blood circulation problems

Through the years, both laboratory research and the practical experiences of surgeons have pointed conclusively to the fact that positive ions have a bad effect on the blood of patients, while negative ions are beneficial.

White blood cells control blood clotting and are normally negatively charged. Because they are of the same charge, they repel each other and do not normally coagulate.

Inhalation of air with an overdose of positive ions causes the white blood cells to lose some of their repelling effect and they become more likely to cling together to form clots, resulting in post-surgery thrombosis.

A recent study carried out in the Conscious Health Clinic in the UK, on the effects of negative ions on blood using the Elanra medical grade negative ion generator, showed that within 20 minutes, blood cells became "less sticky" and they no longer clotted together.

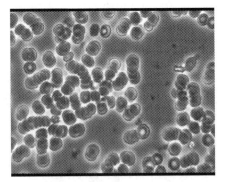

Before breathing ionized air

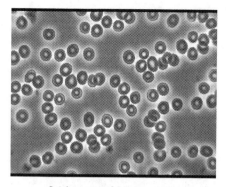

24 hours of ionized air

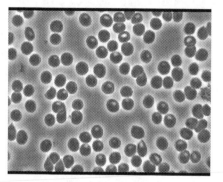

3 weeks of ionized air

Blood samples taken after 24 hours and 3 weeks of breathing negative oxygen ions from the Elanra air ionizer showed that blood cells become significantly less sticky and more oxygenated. Heavily pigmented blood cells indicate the presence of an increased amount of oxygen-carrying hemoglobin.

The effects of high ion concentration on blood circulation have been applied medically in Russia and countries of Eastern Europe. In Hungary, operating theatres and post-surgery recovery wards are commonly equipped with negative ion generators. In Russia, there is widespread use of the negative ion generator in hospitals.

In addition, in some Swiss hospitals, negative ion machines are installed in most delivery and post-delivery rooms. Doctors are under the impression that new mothers are depleted of bioelectric potential. Thrombosis is a threat to women when they have given birth and the negative ions protect against that.

Tests have shown that negative ions in the air help lower the number of deaths during childbirth and help the mother to regain her strength, energy and mental wellbeing. They have also been shown to help lactation.

Negative ions relieve pain

Another scientist, Dr Igho Kornblueh of the American Institute of Medical Climatology in Philadelphia, USA, discovered that exposure to negative ions relieved pain. This institute has been involved in extensive research into negative ions and their effects. Dr Kornblueh proved that patients who were exposed to negative ions within the first one or two days post-surgery felt better and suffered less pain.

On one occasion when a factory worker was rushed to Northeastern hospital with second degree steam burns on his back and legs, Dr Kornblueh intervened. He attached a negative ionizer to the patient's mouth and nose and within minutes the pain was gone. Opiate-based pain medication, usually administered in such cases, was not necessary.

Dr Kornblueh and his colleagues had since used negative ion therapy successfully for burn patients. All burn cases at the hospital were then taken to a windowless, ion filled room. Hospitalized patients were treated for 1 to 1.5 hours a day and outpatients for twenty five to thirty minutes to negative ion concentrations as high as 10,000 ions per cubic centimeter. Within 10 minutes, the pain from the burn had gone. In 85 percent of the patients, no pain medicine needed to be administered. Northeastern's Dr Robert McGowan said, "Negative ions make burns dry out faster, heal faster and with less scarring. They also reduce the need for skin-grafting. They make the patient more optimistic. He sleeps better."

One positive side effect reported by the burns victims to Dr Kornblueh was that the patients with respiratory conditions reported an improvement. Chronic bronchitis and asthma sufferers told him that they could breathe better during and after exposure to the negative ions.

After such positive results with the burn therapy, Dr Kornblueh worked with Dr J R Minehart (Chief Surgeon at Northeastern) and his associate Dr T David to relieve deep, postoperative pain. An eight month long trial period exposed 138 patients to negative ions on the first and second days after surgery.

In 57 per cent (79 cases), the negative ions eliminated or drastically reduced the pain. Dr Minehart said, "At first, I thought it was voodoo. Now I'm convinced that it's real and revolutionary."

Increased levels of serotonin present in damaged tissues causes great pain. As negative ions break down serotonin into a harmless form (5HA; 5-hydroxyindolacetic acid) in the blood and wound area, exposure to negative ions will no doubt decrease pain and consequently the stress level and blood pressure of the patient too.

Adverse drug reactions to medication are the 4th leading cause of death in the US, only behind heart disease, cancer and strokes. Pain management with high concentration of negative ions is safe and natural and reduces the need for dangerous pain medication.

Negative Ions reduce the risks of hospital acquired infections

While working as a microbiologist and experimental pathologist in the department of bacteriology at the University of California, Dr Krueger found that even small amounts of negative ions kill infectious bacteria and quickly take them out of the air. The germ-killing effect of negative ions helps create a clean, bacteria-free atmosphere.

The study referred to in Chapter Five, conducted by the University of Leeds at St James Hospital in the UK, which found that air ionizers wiped out antibiotic resistant aceineobacter from the air, reducing infection rate to zero during the year-long trial, made such an impression on the hospital staff that they wished to retain the ionizers after the study was completed.

Hospitals have become particularly notorious for spreading deadly infections. In the United States, more than two million people are affected by hospital-acquired infections each year, and a whopping 100,000 people die as a result.

The ionizer has become an effective weapon in the fight against hospital acquired infections. Patients requiring hospital stay should bring their own medical grade ionizers to protect themselves while they recover.

Negative ions promote wound healing

In his clinical applications of high negative ion concentration, Dr Kornblueh observed that pain, restlessness and incidence of infection were reduced and healing promoted.

Whether it is a surgical incision, or damaged tissues due to burns or accidents, a high concentration of negative ions aids in the healing process without leaving unsightly scars.

Scars result when wounds do not close up quickly due to repeated and chronic infections caused by exposure to atmospheric bacteria. It is noteworthy that the putrid smell of rotting flesh usually associated with severe burn accidents are absent in cases treated with negative ionization.

Research published in the *Journal of Hygiene* discovered that ionization produced some excellent results when it came to bacteria in burns and plastic surgery units. Levels were reduced by over 96 percent after a two week period—this is remarkable. The healing of patients is greatly improved and very rapid.

Another case study for healing after burns came from Claire Maxwell Hudson, an English television presenter. Claire spilt hot tea on her stomach and suffered second degree burns. This news was distributed over the gossip columns, but several months later, Claire reassured the public by telling of her negative ion machine.

She had bought one prior to the burn to help with her allergies. When she got burnt, she held it to the wound 3 times a day. After two days the pain was gone and after a few weeks there wasn't even a scar. She very happily announced that she'd still be wearing bikinis.

5 Steps to ensuring a quick recovery time and a shorter hospital stay

Step 1) Bring an air ionizer to the hospital

A therapeutic medical-grade air ionizer is a must for post-operative care. Ionizers have been used in hospitals in Europe, Japan and many Russian countries for many years to speed up healing and relieve pain. With the added benefit of killing bacteria in the air, they are no doubt a favorite of doctors. Dr Kornblueh's report from his burn trials in the 1960s also mentioned that there was a 'sedative' and 'tranquilizing' effect on burn patients. An ionizer by the bed invariably results in a feeling of well-being, sounder sleep and a less painful night.

Step 2) Take therapeutic doses of vitamin C

Before going to the hospital, start taking mega doses of vitamin C. Take it throughout the hospital stay and during recuperation for less infection, less pain, quicker healing time, and less bleeding. People who take high doses of vitamin C are much less likely to have blood clotting, inflammation, and other complications.

In the 1940s, Dr Frederick R. Klenner consistently cured chicken pox, measles, mumps, tetanus and polio with the aggressive use of vitamin C. Vitamin C is remarkably safe even in extremely high doses, with virtually no side-effects compared to commonly used prescription drugs.

How much vitamin C is an effective therapeutic dose? Dr. Klenner recommends 350mg per kilogram body weight each day.

Step 3) Take a multivitamin with your meals

Increase your nutritional intake to aid the body's natural healing process. If you are too weak to be chomping down a regular meal, try getting liquidized greens in a smoothie.

A probiotic supplement would also help digestion and assimilation. As with all other supplementation, check with your doctor to see any specific vitamin should not be taken with a particular procedure or medication.

Step 4) Have a friend or family member with you 24 hours a day

Besides having some company and moral support, a guard makes sure that mistakes aren't made, or if mistakes are made, you've got a witness. Preventable medical errors kill and seriously injure hundreds of thousands of Americans every year. So it is ok to question, to make requests and even to appear uncooperative. If the doctor says something you do not understand, ask him/her what it means. It is of great advantage to have a personal advocate who can look out and speak up for you and ensure you are given proper care if you cannot do so yourself.

Step 5) Maintain a happy and optimistic attitude

Psychoneuroimmunology is a field of study on the influence of the brain on the immune system. In this field, doctors and researchers study the links between the mind and health.

Your state of mind strongly influences your immune system. Having a positive and optimistic mind-set may mean a shorter hospital stay.

Qualities like faith, hope, and forgiveness, and the use of social support and prayer also seem to have a noticeable effect on healing.

Results from several studies indicate that people with strong religious and spiritual beliefs heal faster from surgery, are less anxious and depressed, have lower blood pressure, and cope better with chronic illnesses.

One clinical study by US researchers at Duke University Medical Center on 1718 older adults in North Carolina, found that those who attend regular religious services tended to have better immune function.

In another clinical study of 232 older adults undergoing heart surgery, those who were religious were three times less likely to die within six months after surgery than those who were not.

It is true that one does not just suddenly have faith, or a group of supportive people just appear during life's emergencies. Spiritual qualities need to be cultivated and relationships need to be nurtured.

Now is the time to take stock of our lives and attitudes. A critical, negative attitude will bring only unhappiness and isolation. Healing our relationships with God and others often brings physical healing and wholeness.

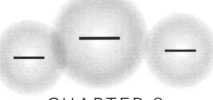

CHAPTER 9

Advice to People with Sleep Problems

"No one can violate Nature's Law and escape her penalties."
—Julian Johnson

Mary had suffered from insomnia for years. She was very familiar with the feeling of being not fully alive.

Every night, no matter what time she went to bed, she would wake up later and could be awake for up to three hours at a time. She discovered that the best time to wake up was 12 midnight, as that gave her the potential to get at least three hours sleep before she had to get up for her job at 7.00 am.

The worst time to wake was at 4.00 am when there was little chance of getting any decent sleep before she had to get up again.

Mary had tried everything. She had been to doctors and tried a variety of pharmaceutical preparations that had been approved by the government for their sleep inducing abilities. They left her feeling hung-over the next day and she did not like the idea of using chemicals to do something that she felt she should be able to do naturally.

Her friends had introduced her to herbal preparations. Sniffing chamomile or drinking chamomile tea did not seem to work and neither did sniffing lavender sachets before bedtime.

Her job was so busy that she could not afford to waste time feeling rotten every day.

Then something amazing happened.

Max, her dog, had always shared her bedroom with her, but just recently he had become a little smelly, as elderly dogs do. Mary disliked this, but at the same time she enjoyed the security that Max's presence offered. She read that she would be able to reduce the doggy smell by placing an ionizer in the room.

Mary purchased a therapeutic ionizer, plugged it in, and hoped it would deal with the doggy smell. That night she had the best sleep that she had ever had. She also noticed that she felt good, which was something that had become almost unfamiliar to her over the years.

Both relieved and puzzled, Mary decided it was time for a bit of internet research. She googled the ionizer and read reviews left by other customers. She noted that several people had commented on the quality of their sleep and how it had improved since they had been using the ionizer.

After years of different medication, years of sleepless nights, years of feeling exhausted and drained throughout the day, Mary had found an extremely simple cure for her insomnia.

Why it is important to get a good night's sleep

It is impossible to have good health without quality sleep. Yet, up to 20 percent of the general population can have trouble falling asleep at night. It is estimated that over 60 million Americans have some type of sleeping issue. For about 40 million people, insomnia is a chronic problem.

Sleep is essential for our wellbeing. Deep restful sleep builds up the body's resistance to diseases, promotes healing and allows for deep physical and mental restoration. It is often observed that poor sleep is followed shortly by a sore throat, a drippy nose or a full blown flu infection.

Serious health problems such as diabetes, stroke, high blood pressure, heart disease, and irregular heartbeats have been linked to sleep deprivation and so has lack of good judgment, weight gain, and psychosis.

Without a good night's sleep, our work productivity and physical appearance will be adversely affected. We cannot perform at our optimum the next day and we can be left looking washed out with a pallid complexion. Lack of sleep ages our skin, leading to wrinkles, dark circles under the eyes and lackluster skin.

Sleep deprivation releases an excess of the stress hormone cortisol, which breaks down collagen reducing skin elasticity. Moreover, without deep restful sleep, the production of the human growth hormone is hampered. This is necessary to help repair body tissues, add muscle mass and thicken the skin to keep us looking youthful.

Good sleep is not only important for our functionality but without it we tend to put on weight as we eat more calories trying to find the energy that we don't have. Sleep loss also seems to stimulate craving for high-fats and high carbohydrate foods and people who sleep less are more likely to become obese.

A survey of over 87,000 adults conducted between 2004 and 2006 by the US National Center for Health Statistics confirmed a link between obesity and sleep loss. One third of those surveyed who slept less than six hours were obese.

With inadequate sleep, we can find ourselves becoming agitated and annoyed faster too. In a study conducted at the University of Pennsylvania in 1997, researchers found that people with inadequate sleep felt stressed, angry, sad and mentally exhausted.

Over time sleeplessness can also contribute to depression, lower libidos and loss of interest in sex—all of which can have an impact on our relationships with our loved ones.

Sleep deprivation is also a big public road safety hazard. Drowsiness slows reaction time, which accounts for up to 100,000 auto crashes per year in the US. Repeated work accidents are also reportedly the result of excessive daytime sleepiness.

Why sleep medication does not work

Insomnia can have many devastating effects on our lives and yet insomniacs often suffer for months or even years, not knowing how to get better and sometimes driven to the point of despair and depression. Some attribute their sleep problem to stress at work and believe that, just like stress, it is something they just have to learn to cope with.

Others turn to over-the-counter drugs or consult a doctor. Some sufferers do not seek treatment for fear that they may be labeled psychotic. They reason that since they are not sick, then they will probably be diagnosed as suffering from a psychological condition. Still others are apprehensive about taking addictive prescriptive medication.

The trouble with pharmaceutical drugs is that they lose their effectiveness over time and patients need larger and larger doses to achieve results. Lunesta, for instance, is the only prescriptive drug approved for long-term usage in the US and has been shown to remain effective for up to six months. Beyond that period, larger doses would be required.

Even if there is some short-term benefit, prescriptive sleep aids do not provide a long-term solution because they do not address the root of the sleep problem. They simply mask the symptoms and perpetuate the problem.

In addition to the usual side effects of sleep medication, grogginess, brain fog, dry mouth and troubling dreams, sleeping pills do not promote deep sleep. Users wake up tired, feeling unrested with headaches and aching muscles. There is also no improvement in work productivity and daytime function.

The root cause of most sleep problems is a messed-up internal body clock

Traditional Chinese medicine constantly stresses the relation of deep sound sleep to health and longevity. "Those who sleep well can eat well and live long."

Deep restful sleep is one of the most pleasurable activities in life. Recall the last time you had a good night's sleep. You were revitalized, refreshed, energized and ready to go. You were unstoppable.

Unless we identify and take active steps in addressing the real cause of our sleep problem, we cannot effectively treat it.

There are several reasons for sleep disorders but most chronic insomniacs are simply "out of sync" with their internal body clock.

Our body temperature rises and falls subtly throughout the day in cycles. This is also known as the circadian rhythm or the internal "sleep clock", which regulates our sleep cycle. Insomniacs have departed from the natural sleep pattern and thrown the body clock out of rhythm. Restoring natural sleep pattern is key to overcoming insomnia.

How to reset our natural sleep pattern

1. Increase exposure to sunlight

The body's natural sleep system is regulated by body temperature, sunlight exposure, and the hormone called melatonin, which controls when and how long we sleep. In nature, we see a variation of this at work in animals that hibernate and sleep through the winter.

The daily cycles of day and night that correlate with the intensity of sunlight affect our body temperature and the level of melatonin in our body. In the day, as our eyes are exposed to sunlight, the melatonin level drops, our body temperature increases, and we feel alert and active.

Conversely, towards the evening as it gets dark, the lack of sunlight causes our melatonin level to increase, followed by a drop in body temperature which induces sleepiness.

Consequently, getting enough sunlight exposure is critical in strengthening our circadian rhythm. Sunlight exposure regulates the natural production of melatonin and helps us sleep better. A very real problem with many of us today is that we do not get enough sunlight exposure, nor do we experience real darkness.

We spend a great part of our day in tightly sealed offices with artificial lighting and after work we live in areas that are very well lit. Our visual senses do not perceive marked differences of day and night and this keeps the melatonin levels from rising and falling within an acceptable range, resulting in sleep disorders.

It makes sense, therefore, to get into the sun as much as possible during the day. If you have to work indoors, make it a point to take breaks and come outside for a breather to receive some intense natural light and refreshing negative ions.

Keep curtains and shades open during the day; move your favorite chair to a sunny spot. If for any reason, you have to be confined indoors for an extended period of time, consider using a light therapy box to simulate daylight.

2. Incorporate an exercise routine

Physical inactivity also contributes to poor sleep. Studies show that more than 50 percent of the people who experience insomnia are inactive, and live a very sedentary lifestyle. The lack of physical activity can contribute to insomnia by inhibiting the daily rise and fall of the body-temperature rhythm.

We have become very removed from our native world. We no longer need to hunt for our food or toil in the fields. Technology and modern gadgets have replaced manual work. In the name of efficiency and productivity, we have succeeded in bringing convenience into our lives with time and energy saving devices such as microwave ovens and remote controls. We have traded physical exertion for constant activity that causes constant stress. Stress will also keep us awake at night.

Physical movement during the day ensures good quality sleep at night. It stimulates a faster temperature rise and regulates our sleep-wake cycle. An exercise program in the morning promotes a quick temperature rise and increases our energy levels so that we are more wakeful, alert and motivated.

Of course there are other great health benefits of physical movement, associated with better blood circulation and deep breathing, as we have seen throughout this book. But a significantly higher peak body temperature in the day due to physical exercise ensures a compensatory dip in temperature in the evening, so that you fall asleep easily, as well as sleep deeply without interruption.

A recent study conducted by Stanford University School of Medicine found that adults who exercise for twenty to thirty minutes every other day by walking or engaging in low impact exercises, are able to fall asleep 50 percent faster and to increase sleep time by almost an hour.

Participants of a recent study by the Feinberg School of Medicine at Northwestern University reported that aerobic exercise resulted in a dramatic improvement in the quality of sleep, including sleep duration. These participants were middle-aged and older adults with a diagnosis of insomnia. They also reported fewer depressive symptoms, more vitality, and less daytime sleepiness.

While still on the topic of exercise, experts who study the connection between physical exercise and longevity said that outdoor exercise demonstrates more health benefits compared with doing the same activities indoors.

Researchers at the University of Exeter in the United Kingdom, who published their review in *Environmental Science and Technology* in 2011 found that exercising outdoors was associated with feeling more revitalized and energetic, and less fatigued, tense, angry or depressed, than after similar indoor activity.

Exercising forces us to breathe deeply so we inhale larger amounts of healthful negative air electricity and exercising outdoor in green spaces naturally doubles up on the rewards. So, for those who will sleep better and longer, take at least 20 minutes of deliberate outdoor time to move and connect with nature in your favorite green space, be it a wilderness area, wildlife reserve or your neighborhood urban park.

How to have a good night's sleep every night

Sleeping disorders and sleep deprivation are afflictions which affect people's attitudes and ability to work and play effectively. However, there are many things we can do to ensure a good night's sleep every night. The following steps would empower us to banish insomnia forever and to enjoy deep, energizing sleep.

Step 1) Balancing our internal clock

Natural sleep researchers assert that energizing sleep can be restored within as little as three days by harmonizing our internal sleep clock. As we have seen, incorporating sun-filled physical activities into our daily routine are steps towards rebalancing our circadian rhythm.

Good health comes from following the natural cycles and rhythms of nature. Those who stay up really late and work deep into the night all the time are hurting their health and rapidly aging their bodies and faces.

Going to sleep and waking up at the same time each day, will condition your body to fall into a routine of sleep and wakefulness. It is best not to disrupt this routine, such as by sleeping in on weekends.

Step 2) Avoid caffeine and other stimulants after twelve noon

Caffeine drinks, including coffee, tea, cola and cocoa are stimulants which cause an adrenalin rush, resulting in increased heartbeat and blood pressure. The body is consequently awoken. Not only are they stimulating, they can be addictive. After the effects of the drink wear off, the body starts to crave it again.

If you enjoy your caffeine beverages, drink them in the morning so that you won't have trouble falling asleep at night. Caffeine can also be found in some ice-cream, yoghurt, chocolate and prescriptive medicine. MSG or monosodium glutamate, a widely used food enhancer, is also a stimulant and should be avoided as it may aggravate insomnia.

Step 3) Induce sleep naturally with brainwave entrainment technologies

Brainwave entrainment or "brainwave synchronization," is any practice that aims to cause brainwave frequencies to fall into step with a periodic stimulus, having a frequency corresponding to the intended brain-state.

Just as soothing music puts us in a state of relaxation while upbeat contemporary music excites us, brainwave entrainment aids can be used safely to induce sleep. Brainwave Entrainment uses sound or images to alter your brainwaves. Your brain state can be shifted to a state of deep rest and sleep simply by shifting these wave patterns.

According to a poll released on March 2, 2009 by the National Sleep Foundation, one-third of Americans lose sleep over the state of the U.S. economy and other personal financial concerns. Brainwave entrainment provides a natural way to shut off such compulsive thinking which seems to turn on automatically whenever our heads hit the pillow.

There are many CDs which use brainwave technology to evoke restful sleep, among which are Dr Ben Kim's "Soft Ocean Dreamland" and Garret LoPorto's "Psychoactive Sounds".

Ion-emitting frequencies of therapeutic negative ion generators have also been proven to be effective as brainwave pattern modulators. Studies conducted at the Brain Development Research Centre by Japanese scientists showed that within two seconds of a leading ion generator being switched on, the brain of a subject one meter away switched to match the frequency emitted by the device.

Negative oxygen ions pulsed at selected frequencies stimulate the brain to respond to and align with these pulses. The brain can then be naturally induced towards the desired brainwave state and its inherent benefits.

A therapeutic air ionizer typically incorporates several ion-emitting frequencies that have been proven to assist sleep by moderating brainwave patterns to promote relaxation at 10Hz or to induce deep sleep at 4Hz.

Programmability is an important feature to look out for in air ionizers. A negative ion generator with a fixed ion frequency of more than 25Hz may keep one alert and awake longer at night than desired. Natural sleep induction through brainwave entrainment does not come with the side-effects of drugs and is safe and non-addictive.

Step 4) Quit Smoking

The old adage "giving up smoking is easy, I have done it a thousand times" is often so true.

Everyone wants to, but something always prevents them from doing it, be it peer pressure from friends while having a social drink or some trigger mechanism such as stress at work.

However, studies have shown that those who quit smoking begin to sleep better almost immediately. Nicotine affects sleep by increasing brain activity, respiration rate and heart rate. Besides the well-known hazards linked with smoking, including emphysema, cancer and stroke, it is addictive and aggravates sleep problems.

There are now many smoking-cessation aids available, such as gums, patches and drugs to help smokers quit the habit. However, these drugs may come with very undesirable side effects. FDA warned that some of these smoking cessation drugs have been linked with serious mental symptoms, including changes in behavior, hostility, agitation, depressed mood and suicidal behavior.

Australian Joshua Shaw has been working in ionization for over forty years and is the renowned inventor of the medical-grade Elanra therapeutic ionizer. He tells how he has helped many people to be completely free of the habit using his air ionizer programmed at 32 Hz—also known as the addiction-reducing frequency.

He himself took only one week to drop from eighty cigarettes a day to zero. "You will experience withdrawal symptoms but by using the ionizer every night and during the day when the need arises, it's a breeze," he said.

Breathing negative ions of oxygen from his ionizer will also induce a detox action such that the nicotine and other nasties are eliminated through the pores in your skin and can stain your mattress bright yellow and brown. Thus, it is advisable to get protection for your mattress. Your skin will also start to take on a fresh appearance and your face will start to glow.

In a recently published report in the journal *Addiction*, British researchers found that exercise may temporarily stop nicotine cravings. Instead of reaching out for the next cigarette when the craving to smoke becomes overwhelming, why not take a jog or a brisk walk or go biking. Engaging in outdoor activity and breathing in charges of electricity might boost your mood, so that you don't feel as great a need to feel better by smoking,

Step 5) Adopt an unprocessed and whole food diet

We have said this several times already in this book, but it cannot be stressed too strongly. A diet comprising of unprocessed organic whole foods ensures that we get the nutrients our body needs for growth, repair and healing without the unhealthful cravings for sugar or other stimulants that interfere with good sleep.

Vitamin B and calcium deficiency, for instance, are factors in insomnia and these are due to overconsumption of refined, nutrients-depleted foods and poor absorption. Allergic reactions due to food and food additives are also known to increase heart rate causing and aggravating insomnia.

Taking vitamin and calcium supplements together with a healthy diet frequently cures sleep disorders and so does reduction in the use of salt and avoidance of allergy-causing foods. Many insomnia sufferers are completely cured by dietary changes alone.

Step 6) Eliminate stored heavy metal from the body

Heavy metal poisoning, such as lead and mercury toxicity, is a documented cause of nervousness, mental confusion and sleep disorder. The use of aluminum-containing drugs such as certain brands of antacids, having new amalgam dental fillings, or disturbing an existing amalgam filling by removing it, using aluminum cooking utensils or aluminum foil in cooking, or even drinking unfiltered water from the tap may result in heavy metal poisoning.

Cases have been recorded where the removal of an amalgam dental filling led to years of sleep problems. Not until the link between the cause and effect was made, and the sufferers started a chelation procedure, were they able to sleep well again.

To treat heavy metal poisoning, Chlorella, a single-cell fresh water algae, has been proven to bind to heavy metals as well as other toxic substances in the bowel and help with the detoxification process.

Zeolite is a naturally occurring mineral, formed from the fusion of lava and ocean water. Liquid Zeolite, such as the Activated Liquid Zeolite supplied by Waiora, has powerful chelation capabilities and is especially useful for detoxifying the human body of carcinogens, heavy metals and viruses. It has been used for more than 800 years in Asia as a remedy for overall health and well-being.

Step 7) Create an environment conducive to sleep

We spend about one third of our lives in our beds. It is during sleep that our strength is renewed and our bodies are rejuvenated for yet another day. There is a Chinese saying, "resting is to prepare to embark on a longer journey", so it makes sense to create a wonderfully relaxing, sleep-inducing environment for deep, refreshing sleep.

* Enliven your sleep environment with negative ions

  The human body is a self-rejuvenating entity with the ability to repair itself during periods of rest and sleep.

  Installing a therapeutic ionizer close to your bed is the best thing that you can do to improve your sleep naturally.

  Abnormal blood levels of serotonin due to poor air quality with high concentration of positively charged air ions in the home or work place has also been shown to lead to insomnia, anxiety and hyperactivity. Exposure to small negative oxygen ions from a medical grade air ion generator has been shown to provide almost instant relief in some cases.

  If you are suffering from pain and as a consequence you are not getting good sleep, the tranquilizing effect of an abundance of negative ions could be what is required to get you back to good health. Inhaling negative ions also boosts the body's immune function, helping the body to fight off diseases and to heal while you sleep. A medical grade air ionizer with programmable functionalities also doubles up as a brain entrainment tool to help induce deep sleep.

- Keep all stress and unnecessary stimulation away from the bedroom

Reserving your bedroom for only sleep and lovemaking will help you unwind and relax as soon as you enter. Turn off all electronic devices. Refuse to be bothered by unfinished work or coming engagements as you settle into bed. Now is also a good time for prayers, thanksgivings and meditation.

- Sleep in complete darkness

This will stimulate the body to produce melatonin to induce sleepiness. Darkness promotes melatonin production whereas light inhibits it. Thus, the darker it is when you sleep, the better your melatonin production, and the better the quality of your sleep.

- Avoid watching TV or using your computer for at least an hour before going to bed. These technologies emit blue light which is quite identical to the natural outdoor light during the day. This tricks your brain into thinking it is still daytime, inhibiting melatonin secretion and perpetuating insomnia.

- Lower the temperature

Create good sleep weather by turning down the air conditioner, turning on the fan and sleeping with less clothing. The cooler the atmosphere, the quicker our body temperature is lowered and the better we sleep.

- Minimize radio frequency radiation and reduce electrical fields

Electromagnetic radiation from electrical appliances and wireless technologies lowers our melatonin levels, which control our immune system in response to cancer and other diseases. Artificial electrical fields will also keep you from sleeping soundly.

The sleep pattern, general behavior and study of a 13-year-old were observed to be getting worse as time went by. A check showed that an electrical clock at his bedhead was emitting a strong electrical field onto his pillow. The clock was removed to a position about 6 feet from the bed. Within a month, he had established a good sleep pattern and his general behavior and study patterns had also normalized.

10-month-old Baby Jones started to have disturbed sleep and would cry a great deal, eventually ending up screaming. A check showed that a 50 Hz radiation was present on the cot pillow.

This came from a battery charger attached to the wall of the adjoining room. The charger to operate a desk calculator was always plugged in and turned on. Within six to eight weeks of relocation to another room, Baby Jones had become a normal and happy child.

Hundreds of case studies surveyed in recent years show conclusively that invisible lines of electric energy play a major part in the pattern of people's health. It is thus prudent to locate such radiations and avoid them where possible.

It is especially important to take breaks from these fields at night when you are sleeping so you can repair and rejuvenate.

Unplug all electrical devices including your bedside lamp and use a battery-operated alarm clock instead of an electric one. Avoid using electric blankets or heating pads.

- Make yourself comfortable

  Finally, make sure your mattress, bedding and sheets are comfortable and inviting. A firm mattress and suitable pillows are necessary for good sleep posture and spinal support. Make sure your bed is also spacious enough for your stature.

Several pages of this book have been devoted to improving your sleep through understanding your cardiac rhythm and creating a calming sleep haven for yourself with invaluable sleep tips which include electrifying the air of your sleep environment.

We have also explored possible causes of sleep disturbances and ways to eliminate the root of the problem. Armed with this knowledge, you can now make positive changes to improving your sleep for a healthier body, more youthful appearance, and above all a sense of well-being.

CHAPTER 10

Regain your Zest & Vitality and Enhance Your Sexual Relationships

"Man is composed of such elements as vital breath, deeds, thoughts and senses."
—The Upanishads

A sales manager was pleasantly surprised by an unexpected side benefit of installing negative ions generators. He noticed that he had felt more alert and energetic after his firm had equipped all its offices with table-top ionizers six months earlier. He had subsequently installed a smaller one in his car as he spent a substantial amount of time travelling to meet clients. He later placed one in his bedroom and was elated with the effect it had on his sex life. "My wife loves it," he said.

Whereas in the past, he had barely any energy left after work for anything except to eat and watch TV, he was now so revitalized that he could have frequent outings and enjoy greater intimacy with his wife. He attested to increased virility and an enhanced marital relationship.

Air electricity can makes you 'sexy'

In Japanese silk farms, air electricity is employed for the very unusual purpose of making silk worms "sexy". Domesticated silkworm moths have been described as "machines devoted to sex" and in high concentration of air ions, not only do the larvae mature into adults earlier, the adults also mate earlier than usual. The silkworms also produce exceptionally soft and luxuriant silk cocoons.

An article in the *Aeroionotherapy Journal* reported that in a series of experiments involving laboratory animals exposed to high levels of negative ions, male animals exhibited increased testicular stimulation and sperm production and female animals showed improved ovulation.

Seemingly, negative air ions support the endocrine function and stimulate the activity of our sexual organs so that males become more fertile and females more fecund. Unhealthy ionization with excessive positive ions on the other hand has the reverse effect.

Modern threats to our fertility and survival

The two perils of modernity to our health, fertility and survival are stress and environmental contamination. The Chinese health authority blames day-to-day pressures and environmental deterioration for the infertility problems of at least a million men in China. Ye Linyang, Director of the Urology Department of Beijing-based 304 Military Hospital, told the Beijing Times in November 2011 that symptoms of male menopause which should appear in men above 60 can now be found in men around 40.

Let's take a closer look at the dangers that are threatening the loss of our sexuality and the survival of our species and see how we can protect ourselves from these assaults. Negative ion therapy has also been proven as an effective support for sexual health.

Stress is the root cause of over 90 percent of all disease

Modern life is full of hassles, deadlines, frustrations and demands. For many people, stress is so commonplace that it has become a way of life. But when you're constantly running in emergency mode, your mind and body pay the price. Chronic stress contributes to heart disease, high blood pressure and strokes. It causes indigestion, suppresses the immune system and upsets hormonal balance. Stress will also adversely affect your sex life.

Unhappiness, tension and anxiety are the greatest fun-killers. Moreover if you have a health condition due to stress, your sexual function will inevitably be compromised. If you are completely sapped of energy, or having difficulty breathing, then you are probably not going to feel sexually stimulating or stimulated. Many incidences of marital break-up stem from unfulfilling sex. Men may blame their wives for their lowered performance and seek out more stimulating partners for reassurance. Women may also attribute their lack of sex drive to an unhappy marriage.

It is essential to manage your stress for a healthier body, greater vitality and happier relationships. We have already devoted an entire chapter, Chapter 4, to ways of reducing and eliminating stress. Here are some more quick tips to beat stress:

- Implement time management methods
- Avoid conflicts at work
- Laugh frequently; we all do silly things sometimes
- Practice relaxation techniques such as deep abdominal breathing and meditation
- Surround yourself with the right kind of air electricity

Negative ion therapies for sexual health

Besides stressful situations, prolonged exposure to bad quality air with severely distorted air electricity also leads to the over secretion of the stress neuro-hormone serotonin, causing many unpleasant symptoms including diminished sex drive.

Stress and breathing bad air both trigger similar internal chemical reactions within the body. Inhalation of fresh air with an abundance of negative ions on the other hand, has the reverse effect.

It promotes relaxation by increasing the conversion of serotonin into a harmless, inactive metabolite (5-HT), imparting a sense of well-being.

Furthermore, as we saw above, negative ions stimulate the activities of the sexual organs, heightening sexual pleasure, enhancing male potency, and increasing the chance of conception. They make us "sexy".

Pregnancy and miscarriage

A study carried out by Dr Sulman in the 1950s recognized that women who were subjected to an overload of serotonin will abort their babies. This means that being pregnant but dealing with too much stress or too many positive ions will more than likely result in a miscarriage.

Dr Sulman's experiments involving pregnant rats showed that they abort if injected with serotonin. Later he worked with twenty women undergoing legalized abortion who subsequently lost their pregnancies when given drugs to induce artificial overproduction of serotonin.

He also observed that in some women, the stress involved in trying to have babies and fearing failure causes the over production of serotonin, resulting in unsuccessful pregnancies. In the late 1950s and early 1960s he treated more than a hundred women with recurrent miscarriages with drugs that blocked the natural serotonin production. As a result, almost all of these 'habitual aborters', became mothers with healthy babies.

As we have seen earlier in the book, besides the stress of daily living, serotonin overproduction is stimulated by excessive positive atmospheric ions. Unhealthy air electricity in the home or workplace may boycott an otherwise successful pregnancy. And for those who have repeatedly tried and failed to conceive or carry a pregnancy through full term, the "electricity" of your love nest should perhaps be the first place to look into.

Negative ions and lactation

New mothers may experience feelings of anxiety and hopelessness if they are not able to produce enough milk for their new-born. As a result they lose confidence in breastfeeding their babies and turn quickly to milk formulations for the nourishment of their young.

While breastfeeding may require some hard work and persistence, it does help to have some kind of support, such as a nanny, a counselor and a happy, relaxed, electrically charged atmosphere.

Improved ionization with negative ion generators installed in delivery wards of some Swiss hospitals regularly helps new mothers to significantly increase their milk secretion.

A systematic study by Russian ion scientists on the effect of negative ions on lactation showed that women who were unable to breastfeed their babies were able to do so happily after undergoing negative ion therapy.

Prevalence of environmental hormone disruptors

We all know what hormones do. They make men masculine and women feminine. They make us fertile, support pregnancy, give us pimples and cause us to be attracted to the opposite sex.

Testosterone and estrogen are hormones with pivotal roles in sexual performance and fertility. They dictate when we start developing breasts or producing sperm. Testosterone is produced in relatively high amounts in men compared to women, while the reverse is true of estrogen.

In recent years, however, we have seen high incidences of hormone disruption and rising infertility rates. Increasing numbers of little girls are reaching puberty as young as seven years of age.

The American Medical Association estimates that 43 percent of the female population suffers from lack of libido. Sperm counts in men have dropped in the last 50 years. This was reported in the British Medical Journal in 1992 based on a series of 61 studies in semen analysis involving 15,000 healthy men from 20 countries and seven continents.

And according to a report by the European Science Foundation, at least one in every five men in Europe aged 18-25 is considered to be infertile. Birth rates in industrialized nations have fallen dramatically over the past several decades.

Generally, worldwide, it is estimated that one in seven couples have problems conceiving. Breast cancers, infertility, early miscarriages, and falling sperm production in men are signs that our hormonal systems are being hijacked by common but hidden environmental factors.

Human beings are not the only victims. The modern world is also exacting a toll on its wildlife populations. There are increasing observations showing major changes in male reproductive functions in wild animals due to environmental toxins.

Male polar bears in the Arctic regions are being born with both male and female genitalia, impairing reproduction. Male largemouth bass caught in the polluted waters of Potomac River in the US showed female characteristics, some even producing eggs.

Contamination of Lake Apopka in Florida with chemical insecticides in 1980 led to male alligators having underdeveloped genito-urinal organs such that mating was impossible. Florida panthers have low sperm counts, and a high proportion of abnormal sperm cells.

These effects were associated with the presence of environmental pollutants with estrogenic activity in the diet of these animals.

Certain environmental toxins, called endocrine-disrupting chemicals are causing a great deal of sexual and reproductive problems in both wildlife and the human race.

This class of chemicals, also known as "estrogen mimics" or "xeno-estrogens" disrupt the natural hormones in the bodies when ingested causing reproductive irregularities in both animals and humans such as low sperm counts, early puberty and deformed sexual organs.

These chemicals resemble the female hormone estrogen and when they get into the bloodstream, send feminizing signals to the tissues of the body. These estrogen mimickers lower the testosterone level in men, causing them to lose their libido, became impotent, have low sperm counts and increase their risk for prostate diseases.

Xeno-estrogens are also dangerous for women causing them to put on weight, have painful menstruation and become more susceptible to breast and ovarian cancers. They also wreak havoc with the emotions, causing depression and irritability.

The really alarming news is that these foreign estrogen are everywhere and we are exposed to them on a daily basis. They include PCBs (polychlorinated biphenyls); BPA (bisphenol A); phthalates (polyvinyl chloride); the insecticides DDT (dichloro-diphenyl-trichloroethane), PFOA (perfluorooctanoic acid), endosulfan, kepone, dieldrin, methoxychlor, toxaphene and parabens (a chemical preservative used commonly in skin and body products and cosmetics).

These chemicals are found in a wide range of consumer products—plastic toys, sunscreens, pesticides, detergents, Teflon cookware, hair sprays, and even in our food and water supplies.

Of great concern is the prevalence of plastic in our environment. Estrogenic chemical compounds used in the manufacture of plastic leach into our food and water contained in plastic boxes and bottles. Food cans are also lined with estrogen mimicking compounds contaminating the food with excess hormone disruptors. Animal feeds contain dangerous additives including antibiotics, hormones and hormone mimickers to fatten up livestock.

However, no matter how contaminated our environment has become, there are simple ways to safeguard our sexuality and to protect the yet unborn generation. We can limit our exposure to harmful environmental hormone disruptors and enhance our reproductive health by following these steps:

Step 1) Choose organic produce, grown without chemical pesticides

If you cannot get organic, make sure you wash your vegetables thoroughly and remove the peels of your fruits to minimize exposures.

Step 2) Reduce the use of plastics

Store food in glass or ceramic containers. Stainless steel water bottles are also safer than plastic ones as most plastic bottles and containers contain toxins like parabens and BPA that can affect your hormone levels. Do not microwave convenience food in plastic boxes.

Step 3) Buy only grass-fed or hormone free meats

If you get meat from other sources, trim off the fat. Toxic chemicals including estrogen mimickers are stored in the fats of animals

Step 4) Use a water filter

Use a high-quality filter to remove pesticides and other chemical compounds from your drinking water

Step 5) Use organic skin-care products

Avoid skin care products and cosmetics containing parabens, artificial fragrance and phthalates. There are many safer alternatives available, made from organic ingredients that can provide effective protection, coverage as well as nourishment for the skin.

Step 6) Consume more estrogen fighting foods

The estrogen fighting foods are, for example, the cruciferous vegetables: broccoli, cauliflower, brussel sprouts and cabbage, which help with the excretion of excess estrogen.

Step 7) Use an air ionizer to remove airborne chemicals

The ambient air in most indoor environments contains chemicals, volatile organic compounds (VOCs) and other toxins that are often off-gassing from construction materials, paints, furniture, detergents and scented products.

As a bonus, an atmosphere rich in negative ions also help to neutralize the effect of stress hormones, so that we are relaxed and energized for the more important things in life.

Step 8) Increase your intake of foods with natural estrogen inhibiting properties

Fortunately many of these are the delicious things in life. They include berries, citrus fruits, pineapples, pears, grapes, figs, melons, squash, onions, green beans, cabbage, sesame seeds, and pumpkin seeds.

Step 9) Consume more leafy greens

Leafy greens are rich in folate, a vitamin which not only improves fertility in women and ensures the healthy development of fetuses but also helps men with the production of healthy sperm. A study showed that men with low levels of folate have higher percentage of defective sperm.

As an alternative to leafy greens, supplement your diet with folic acid to improve both female and male reproductive health. Royal jelly is also a deeply nourishing food supplement known to enhance fertility. Zinc and anti-oxidants have also proven to help men stay virile well into their advanced years and support optimum prostate health.

Step 10) Relax and de-stress

And if you are following all these tips, together with those in Chapter 4 on eliminating stress, you will find it much easier to relax and enjoy life.

Being fruitful is the most natural thing in the world

The problems that confront us today were the solutions man implemented for yesterday's problems. DDT, for instance, was touted as a breakthrough in modern progress and its developer, Paul Muller was awarded the Nobel Prize in 1948. It was a wonder working miracle, killing crop-destroying pests and malaria-carrying mosquitoes, saving countless lives.

However, it was not until DDT and other hormone disrupting chemicals had been on the market for decades that we began to understand the intricacies of the hormone signaling system within our bodies. Even though it seemed non-threatening to humans at that time, it had begun to attack the foundations of life.

So the bottom line is to return to nature. Eat unadulterated foods that are grown according to nature's design, drink and breathe as nature intended us to. The price of modern conveniences is way too high if we have to pay for them with our lives and the lives of our children.

Our children are coming into an increasingly hostile and unnatural world where even well-meaning parents, the people that are most important to these newcomers, have lost their instinct of how to care properly for their new offspring.

Health care and child care have become so complicated that we are no longer confident in caring for ourselves and our family. As such we delegate this difficult task to qualified medical professionals and organizations.

However, our existing healthcare systems are flawed, with too great a dependence on drugs and chemical medication. We hear all too frequently of medical misadventures that affect hundreds of people every year.

We should rediscover ourselves by going back to nature and reconsider the folk wisdoms that have been passed down from generations, bearing in mind that humans have come a long way living off nature alone.

CHAPTER 11

Say Goodbye to Disease and Get Younger

"Oxygen is the main nutrient of the body. When we improve our oxygen intake, we enhance our immune system and the body's ability to detoxify and stay healthy."
—Dr Michael Schachter, Columbia University.

In her book *Superpower Breathing for Super Energy*, Dr Patricia Bragg told of her father's expeditions to India where he found holy men in secluded unspoiled retreats who spent many hours daily in the practice of deep breathing to build physically powerful bodies as instruments for spiritual advancement. He met a 126-year-old holy man in the foothills of the Himalayan Mountains who had perfect vision, a beautiful head of hair, all his teeth and the endurance and stamina of an athlete. Lifelong deep breathing of fresh air had also kept his skin and muscle tone ageless.

Mr Bragg also met a beautiful 86 year old woman who looked half her age. Apparently, the secret to her agelessness and grace was the perfected art of deep breathing and meditation. These people owed their great strength and mentality and youthfulness to the oxygen-ions rich air which they breathed on a daily basis.

Researchers are now able to prove mathematically that when the level of air pollution decreases by 10 micrograms per cubic meter, then life expectancy for that area increases by more than seven months. From the centenarians of the remote Japanese island of Okinawa, to those of the island of Dominica in the Caribbean and Azerbaijan in Talysh Mountains, fresh air and conscious deep breathing are the secrets to living beyond a hundred years.

Cancer is a modern disease

Recently, a team of researchers from Manchester University, led by Professor Michael Zimmerman and Professor Rosalie David, examined hundreds of mummified bodies, fossil records and classical medical literature and found no sign of cancer except for one isolated case.

With data from historical sources spanning three thousand years, the scientists concluded that cancers must indeed have been rare in ancient times. Cancer is a modern disease caused by environmental factors such as pollution and diet.

The University of Manchester study also indicates that it was not until the 17th century that the first reports of cancer appeared in scientific studies. Alarmingly, the rate of cancer occurrence has risen dramatically during the 20th Century and today, according to the American Cancer Society, 41 percent of all adults will develop cancer in their lifetime.

Other industrialized nations are also not spared from the scourge of this disease. In China, cancer has become the nation's biggest killer. In 2007, the disease was responsible for one in five deaths, an increase of 80 percent since the start of economic reforms 30 years earlier.

Evidently, cancer-causing factors are rampant in modern, industrialized societies. Air pollution, sick buildings, unhealthy food and stressful, profit-driven lifestyles all contribute to the meteoric rise of cancer.

During the presentation of her findings to a group of UK oncologists, Professor David said, "There is nothing in the natural environment that can cause cancer. So it has to be a man-made disease, down to pollution and changes to our diet and lifestyle." And if it is man-made then it is preventable.

Chronic oxygen deprivation is the cause of cancers and other degenerative diseases

Breathing unhealthy, ion-deficient air consistently can cause serious imbalances that lead to cancers and other degenerative diseases.

Dr Kruger demonstrated this many years ago, when creating an environment devoid of negative ions resulted in the demise of his laboratory mice.

Even earlier, Russian scientists had conducted numerous experiments involving raising small healthy animals in air totally depleted of ions. Within two weeks all the animals had died from their inability to utilize oxygen properly without air ions.

The traditional assumption that oxygen alone is the prerequisite for the sustenance of life is flawed. Negative ions are necessary for the absorption of oxygen into the blood stream. Without ions we cannot assimilate oxygen in quantities needed to live.

Through the process of respiration, the body uses oxygen to produce energy. Since our body runs on energy, the lower the level of air ions, the lower the efficiency of our minds and bodies.

Compromised air due to pollution and unnatural living conditions in our cities makes it impossible for us to take in enough oxygen our bodies need for optimal health. This is aggravated by the fact that we do not always remember to breathe deeply throughout the day.

Aerobic and anaerobic respiration

Basic biology tells us that cells typically create energy via a process known as aerobic respiration. Healthy cells are aerobic.

That is to say they function properly in the presence of sufficient oxygen. They metabolize or "burn" oxygen and blood sugar to produce packets of energy (ATP) which are needed for basic cellular activities such as cell repair and the manufacture of proteins, enzymes, hormones and neurotransmitters.

Carbon dioxide, which is the by-product of this energy making process, is used to extract oxygen from hemoglobin, the red blood cells that transport oxygen from the lungs to the cells. This energy creating cycle within the body continues indefinitely. It is also called the Krebs cycle, after the Nobel laureate Hans Krebs who first identified the cycle in 1937.

However, if the blood's ability to transport oxygen is inhibited, or the amount of oxygen is lowered, or the cells are prohibited from absorbing oxygen from the blood, then the Krebs cycle is disrupted.

All these can happen if the air that we breathe is chronically ion-depleted. When a cell does not get enough oxygen, it has no energy. A survival mechanism kicks in and the cell changes to anaerobic respiration. The cell stops depending on oxygen and starts fermenting blood sugar to make energy.

Lactic acid, a waste product of that fermentation process further deprives the cell of oxygen. According to health researcher and chemist, Dr David Gregg, "Cancer does not cause cells to turn anaerobic but rather it is stabilized anaerobic respiration that is the single cause that turns the normal cells that depend on aerobic respiration into cancer cells."

A well-oxygenated body cannot accommodate disease germs

Optimal oxygenation of our body is the secret to keeping us youthful and disease-free. Natural doctors have asserted that the primary cause of all diseases is linked in one way or another to oxygen deficiency. A well oxygenated body is extremely hostile to disease germs.

In 1931, Dr Otto Warburg won the Nobel Prize in Physiology for proving that viruses cannot proliferate or exist in a highly-oxygenated environment. This is due to the fact that viruses are anaerobic; that is, they thrive in the absence of oxygen.

He stated that the prime cause of cancer is oxygen deprivation at the cellular level, and cancer cells cannot survive in an oxygen-rich environment.

A weakened immune system occurs when the human body lacks oxygen, thereby allowing pathogenic microbes to breed. On the other hand, a highly oxygenated body is a less hospitable environment for opportunistic microbes.

We have seen how negative ion generators are useful as air cleaners, since germs and viruses are destroyed upon contact with negative ions. We have also learnt that even anti-biotic resistant bacteria do not stand a chance against negative ions and are completely eliminated in hospital trials using air ionizers.

Internally, when negative ions are ingested through inhalation, they enable oxygen to be delivered throughout the body, increasing tissue oxygen levels and killing disease causing microorganisms.

Normal cells, however, which depend on oxygen for optimum function and viability, thrive and become healthier. Because of an increase in the oxygen supply, the immune system is boosted, thereby enabling the body to ward off diseases and heal itself.

Ionization therapy

You can effectively increase your oxygen intake by simply breathing air with an abundance of negative ions. Oxygenating the body through ionization therapy can be effected with a therapeutic, medical-grade air ionizer.

In the 1950s, negative ions were produced by harnessing the steady decay of the potentially dangerous radioactive isotope tritium, and it worked very well for scientific studies, producing wonderful results as reported. However, tritium is so dangerous that it is illegal except in fusion power plants and subsequently the tritium machines were seized by the FDA.

Since the 1950s, manufacturers have produced dozens of ion generators for laboratory and home use. Some of these newer generators produce ions using electrostatic, incandescent and ultraviolet means, and the ions deteriorate quickly. In addition, electrostatic and ultraviolet machines also produce ozone.

More recent advances in electronics have enabled the manufacture of safe, compact machines. An electronic circuit was developed using capacitors and diodes and this system is used in all modern ionizers. However, the new ionizers that were mass-produced in the 1970s failed to live up to expectation. Any apparent beneficial effects they had soon stopped.

Why negative ion generators don't work

Size Does Count

In reviewing the work of earlier researchers, Australian inventor Joshua Shaw came to the conclusion that it was the size of negative ions that was crucial in positively affecting living organisms, including humans.

Not all ions are the same size. There are small, medium and large ions. However, only small negative ions like those found in nature have a positive biological effect on living things.

The first ionizers replicated the natural ion generation process through the decay of radioactive trace substances on the Earth's crust. When inhaled, nature's ions enter the bloodstream, improve respiration and increase overall energy and vitality.

Joshua Shaw discovered that the new machines generated only large negative ions that will eradicate pollutants from the air but have absolutely no positive health effect. In other words, they cannot enter the body to do their good work and are effective only as air-cleaners.

Mass spectrometers were used to discover the speed of biologically active ions found in nature. Small negative ions have a speed of 1.9 square centimeter volts per second. It was discovered that the speed at which ions are produced governs their size. Unless that speed is achieved, only large or medium size ions are produced. They cannot be breathed in, and therefore simply keep the air clean.

Small negative ions of oxygen are not easy to produce by mechanical means. However, the first effective, medically certified ion generator was developed after years of scientific research at Universities, including La Trobe in Melbourne, and the ANU in Canberra, involving collaborative work with all the world's leaders in the field, including research pioneers Albert Krueger, Walter Stark, Igho Kornblueh of the University of Pennsylvania, Felix G Sulman of Israel, C.A. Laws, and Robert Beck, the father of electro medicine.

This first medical grade ionizer incorporates a patented technology that generates biologically active small negative ions of oxygen.

The air ionizer is the missing link in modern living

In recent years, we have seen an increasing application of the benefits of air ionization.

In July 2009, electronics giant LG unveiled a new refrigerator that uses negative ion technology to keep food fresher for longer. After seven days, food stored in the new fridge has more than five times less fungi than in conventional fridges.

The Lexus hybrid luxury car HS250h unveiled at the 2009 Detroit Motor Show also uses negative ion technology to produce air with an equal ratio of positive and negative ions to stop the propagation of airborne germs, mold and bacteria in the cabin.

Research by electronics company Sharp has also shown that positive and negative ions produced by their air conditioning systems can inactivate viruses including influenza.

We can expect to see more of the biggest companies in the world unveil remarkable new applications for negative ion technology to meet the growing consumer demand for healthier, cleaner and greener lifestyles.

Finally, people are starting to realize that negative ionizers are the missing link to a modern, healthier way of life.

However, this book also serves to warn consumers of the emergence of inferior ionizing imitations which will not only disappoint buyers, but adversely affect the credibility of ionization as a reputable and effective therapy.

8 things to consider when shopping for an air ionizer

Here is a comprehensive list of things to look out for when choosing an air ionizer to create a better indoor climate for improved health and wellbeing.

1) Medical certification

Go for machines that are independently endorsed by relevant medical and health authorities for safety and therapeutic purposes. This will ensure that you and your family receive the full benefits of air ionization necessary for your wellbeing.

A medical grade air ionizer supplies an abundance of ingestible, highly charged small oxygen molecules that not only clear the air of pollutants and disease pathogens, but also help to balance the internal body chemistry to boost the immune system and promote healing.

2) No ozone and other toxic by-products

Many so-called air ionizers produce ozone, and other undesirable by-products such as ions of nitrous oxides, which will make us sicker or create other health issues. Ozone, a toxic oxygen allotrope, is useful for sterilizing the air but is dangerous when inhaled.

3) Compliance with all electrical and safety standards

A device that produces air that is to be breathed into the body must be built to a stringent quality assurance standard. Air undergoes metabolic chemical reactions in the body and a machine producing air must be built to the highest standards.

4) RoHS Product Certification

Compliance with the European Directive on the Restriction of Hazardous Substances (RoHS) ensures that the ionizing device is made from materials that do not outgas. Toxic chemical outgassing will add to the discomfort of allergy sufferers.

5) Measurements of ion density

A medical grade air ionizer will produce sufficient quantities of small negative air ions to balance the body and produce beneficial health effects. As a guide, ion concentration of about 250 000 negative ions per cubic centimeter of air has been found to be helpful for relief of asthma symptoms and 350 000 for hay fever and allergies.

However different measurements of ion density are used by different manufacturers of air ionizers and the majority of people do not understand the differences.

For instance, concentration of ions is usually measured in units of cc (cubic centimeters). However some manufacturers measure in units of cm (cubic meters). This is misleading because people understand 'cm' as 'centimeters', and there are 1 000 000 ccs (cubic centimeters) in 1 cm (cubic meter). A machine that generates 300 000 negative ions per cm, effectively produces only 0.3 per cc, and that is why they do not work!

Still other manufacturers measure in ions emitted per second, which is not a real measurement at all because an ionizer might emit millions of ions per second, but they cluster around the machine and go nowhere. The power of an ionizer is not an important factor. It is the ability of the ions produced to travel from the ionizer to the person being treated.

As long as the ions produced are small, like those we find in nature, this will be achieved. Small negative ions are very active—scientists describe them as "zig-zagging around at great speed". They are inhaled to enter the bloodstream through the lungs to exert a biological effect.

Medium to large negative ions, on the other hand, are sluggish and slow moving and merely clean the air.

6) Programmability

The ion density and ion emission frequency of an air ionizer should be adjustable so that it can be programmed to support different health requirements.

The optimal ion concentration for therapeutic purposes differs for different individuals and thus programmability is an essential feature.

While an adult would benefit greatly in an atmosphere with ion concentration of 350 000 negative ions per cc, a baby would fare better in one with just 50 000.

Depending on a user's needs, the ion emission frequency should also be configurable to induce brainwave changes to aid sleep, relaxation, healing or alertness. There are also stabilizing frequencies known to support pain management and one to overcome addictions such as alcoholism, obesity or smoking.

7) ELF fields

Artificial electrical fields pose possible health risks by interfering with the cellular and metabolic functions of the human body. An air ionizer, being a therapeutic device for healing, should not produce ELF levels above the proposed US EPA standard for ELF exposure of 1 milliGauess at 40cm from the device.

Air filtration technology incorporated in many conventional air purifiers employs the use of strong motors to suck air through a series of filters. Having a motor on continuously is not a good idea because high ELF fields are generated. Machines that both ionize and filter the air may also be self-defeating as ions are sucked into the filters rather than being propagated throughout the air to be breathed in.

Large quantities of small, highly mobile negative ions from a medical grade air ionizer can effectively clean the air of pollutants and disease germs without the need for further filtering processes.

Conclusion

It is now clear that in our high consumption throwaway society, we have been polluting the planet. We have polluted our own life-breath, and we have to breathe it back again, resulting in all sorts of ailments, including immune deficiencies and cancers. The technology-rich environment we've created destroys the air we breathe. We can't turn back the clock, but we can start making wise lifestyle choices, and we can use technology to help restore the air that we breathe.

A medical grade air ionizer can help protect us from the ravages of rapid technological advances and help us ensure efficient blood oxygenation. Whenever possible, retreat to the tranquility and beauty of nature and remember the God who freely gives us of the abundance of the Earth. It is in nature that we find healing for our body, mind and soul. And in restoring Nature's air electricity into our environment, we reclaim our life's breath and birth-right which is to have a long and happy life.

People throughout the ages have been looking for the elusive Elixir of Youth. However, it is not going to be a pill or a herb. We have to return to the ways of nature. We will not be indefinitely young, but we can be always youthful. We can all gain inspiration from the words of raw food guru David Wolfe in his video filmed in the untrampled nature of the Hawaiian Island chain. He is enjoying such a great sense of wellbeing that he wants to live three lives in his one life.

My wish is that you too can celebrate health and goodness each moment as you live a full and vibrant life, having the breath of life which is the essence of fresh air, around and in you, and pulsating through every vein.

THE INFORMATION IN
THIS BOOK HAS BEEN SOURCED FROM

The research papers of Bionic Products Pty Ltd (Australia)

Hawkins LH. Air ions and Office Health. Building Services & Environmental Engineer, April, 1981.

Hawkins LH. Problems of Air Ions and Air Conditioning, Human Biology and Health, University of Surrey, Building Services & Environmental Engineer, August, 1979.

Jukes J, Jenkins A, Laws J. Impact of Improved Air Quality on Productivity and Health in the Workplace. Presented at the Healthy Buildings Symposium, Lisbon, June, 2006.

Tchijevsky AL. Transaction of Central Laboratory Scientific Research on Ionification. The Commune, Voronej, 1933.

Krueger AP, Sobel D. Air Ions and Health: chapter in Ways of Health (Holistic Approaches to Ancient and Contemporary Medicine) (Ed.) Sobel, DS. Harcourt Brace Jovanovich, New York, 1979.

Williams P. Obituary: Coppy Laws; Developer of radar and the air ioniser, The Independent, London, 2002, June 4.

Krueger AP et al. Air ion action on bacteria. Int J Biometeor, March 1975;19(1).

Seo KH et al. Bactericidal effects of negative air ions on airborne and surface Salmonella enteritidis from an artificially generated aerosol. USDA/ARS Southeast Poultry Research Laboratory, Athens, Georgia, 2001; 64(1):113-6.

Mitchell BW, Daniel J. Application of negative air ionisation on airborne transmission of Newcastle Disease Virus, King Avian Dis, 1994, Oct-Dec;38(4):725-32.

Sulman, F. G. "Effects of Hot Dry Desert Winds (Sharav, Hamsin) on the Metabolism of Hormones." Journal of the Medical Association of Israel, 1962

Kerr KG et al. Air ionisation and colonisation/Infection with Methicillin-resistant Staphylococcus Aureus and Acinetobacter species in an intensive care unit, Inten Care Med 2006 Feb;32(2):315-7. Epub 2006, Jan 24.

Air Ions And Health by Albert P Kruger and David S Sobel

Back to the Earth by Dr Sydney A, Baggs

The Ion Effect by Fred Soyka with Alan Edmonds

The Ion Miracle by Jean-Yves Cote

ABCs of Asthma, Allergies & Lupus by F. Batmanghelidj, M.D.

Healing the New Childhood Epidemics, Autism, ADHD, Asthma & Allergies by Kenneth Bock, M.D.

Callous Disregard by Andrew J. Wakefield

The Vitamin Cure for Children Health's Problems by Ralph Campbell, M.D., & Andrew W. Saul

The Allergy & Asthma Cure by Fred Pescatore, M.D.

Hormone Deception, D. Lindsey Berkson

Our Stolen Future, Theo Colborn, Dianne Dumanoski, John Peterson Myers

How to Beat the Bird Flu by Mike Adams

End Insomnia Forever and Enjoy Energizing Sleep in as little as 3 Days by Kacper Postawski

The Effects of Air Quality on the Serotonin Irritation Syndrome by Charles Wallach. Ph.D.

Electromagnetic Frequencies: Blog of Dr. Aurelie Laurence, Certified Quantum Biofeedback Specialist. http://cellphonesafety.wordpress.com

Ions Can Do Strange Things to You by Robert O'Brian, the Rotarian

2007 BioInitiative Report: A Rationale for a Biologically-based Public Exposure Standard for Electromagnetic Fields (ELF and RF); http://www.bioinitiative.org

Application of Negative Air Ionization for Reducing Experimental Airborne Transmission of Salmonella Enteritidis to Chicks, Richard. Gast, 1 Bailey W. Mitchell, and Peter S. Holt

Effect of Negative Air Ionization on Airborne Transmission of Newcastle Disease Virus, Bailey W. Mitchell and Daniel J. King

http://ritalinsideeffects.net/

Lavie, P. Accident Analysis and Prevention, August 1982; vol 14.

Yang PY, Ho KH, Chen HC, Chien MY 'Exercise training improves sleep quality in middle-aged and older adults with sleep problems: a systematic review.' School and Graduate Institute of Physical Therapy, College of Medicine, National Taiwan University, Taipei, Taiwan.

Matthew P. Buman, PhD., 'As people become less active, they have also become less healthy. In 2003, the World's Heart Federation warned that lack of exercise is as bad as smoking a packet of cigarette every day.' Department of Medicine, Stanford University School of Medicine, Stanford, California, mbuman@stanford.edu

Abby C. King, PhD., 'Exercise as a Treatment to Enhance Sleep' Department of Health Research and Policy Stanford Prevention Research Center, Stanford University School of Medicine, Stanford, California

"Chantix and Zyban to Receive Boxed Warnings for Serious Neuropsychiatric Symptoms." Medscape Today (www.medscape.com), 7/1/09.

"Suicide Warnings for 2 Anti-Smoking Drugs." The New York Times (www.nytimes.com), 7/1/09.

FACEMIRE, C.; GROSS, T. & GUILLETTE, L., 1995. Reproductive impairment in the Florida panther: Nature or nurture. Environmental Health Perspectives, 103:79-86.

GUILLETTE, L.; GROSS, T.; MASSON, G.; MATTER, J.; PERCIVAL, H. & WOODWARD, A., 1994. Developmental abnormalities of the gonad and abnormal sex hormone concentrations in juvenile alligators from contaminated and control lakes in Florida. Environmental Health Perspectives, 102:680-688.

The Purest Place On Earth, Dr AL Sears, Power for Healthy Living http://www.alsearsmd.com

http://www.cdc.gov/nchs/fastats/asthma.htm

'Exercise may temporarily ease cigarette cravings' in Medline Plushttp://www.nlm.nih.gov

"The UCLA Population Studies of CORD:. X. A Cohort Study of Changes in Respiratory Function Associated with Chronic Exposure to SOx, NOx, and Hydrocarbons," Am. J. Public Health, vol. 81, no.3, 1991, pp.350-359.

'School Shootings and Psychiatric Drugs' by CEGANT on MARCH 2, 2012 http://cegant.com/commentary/school-shootings-and-psychiatric-drugs

'More than a million men sterile in China' http://europe.chinadaily.com.cn/china/2011-11/07/content_14064887.htm

'Cancer is purely man-made' say scientists after finding almost no trace of disease in Egyptian mummies By FIONA MACRAE http://www.dailymail.co.uk/sciencetech/article-1320507/Cancer-purely-man-say-scientists-finding-trace-disease-Egyptian-mummies.html

Cold weather DOESN'T increase the risk of a heart attack - you're more likely to die from one during winter wherever you are: http://www.dailymail.co.uk/health/article-2229294/Cold-weather-DOESNT-increase-risk-heart-attack--youre-likely-die-winter-are.html#ixzz2HYvEqTYe

Duke Study: Attending Religious Service May Improve Immune Status http://www.
dukehealth.org/health_library/news/663

Spirituality - Trihealth http://trihealth.adam.com/content.aspx?productId=107&pid=33
&gid=000360

Protective and lethal effects of unipolar air ions on microorganisms; Dr A.P.Krueger,
Mr W. Wesley Hicks and Mr J.C. Beckett (U.S.A.) "International Society of
Bioclimatology and Biometeorology" First Bioclimatological Congress Vienna, 23-
27 September 1957

No Mast: Phone Masts and Cancer Clusters http://www.nomasts.org/index.
php?option=com_content&view=article&id=74&Itemid=116

EMR Stop: Phone Mast dangers http://emrstop.org/index.php?option=com_
content&view=category&layout=blog&id=22&Itemid=21

Cancer active: How safe is our modern communication technology? http://www.
canceractive.com/cancer-active-page-link.aspx?n=1540

The Telegraph: Mobile mast blamed for cancer cluster http://www.telegraph.co.uk/
health/healthnews/7567060/Mobile-mast-blamed-for-cancer-cluster.html

World Health Organization/International Agency for Research on Cancer (2011,
May 31). Cell phones and cancer: Assessment classifies radiofrequency
electromagnetic fields as possibly carcinogenic to humans. ScienceDaily.
Retrieved January 15, 2013, from http://www.sciencedaily.com/releases/
2011/05/110531133115.htm

Obituary: Coppy Laws; Developer of radar and the air ionizer. The Independent
(London, England)

Upper respiratory tract infection is reduced in physically fit and active adults http://
www.ncbi.nlm.nih.gov/pubmed/21041243

Shift Work Disorder News http://www.shiftworkdisorder.com/about

Treatment of seasonal affective disorder with a high-output negative ionizer http://www.ncbi.nlm.nih.gov/pubmed/9395604

The Effects of the ELANRA on Brain Waves http://www.elanra.co.uk/brainwaves.htm

ELECTROMAGNETIC FIELDS AND YOUR HEALTH by John Iovine, From "Popular Electronics" March 1993

ABOUT THE AUTHOR

Rosalind Tan, homeschooling mum and elementary school teacher turned health researcher, educator and entrepreneur, runs a business that deals with cutting edge air restoration technologies. This enterprise brings her into close working relations with prominent ion scientists of our time and offers her opportunities to learn from the experts.

rosalind@truthaboutairelectricity.com